MAVERICKS, MIRACLES, AND MEDICINE

The Pioneers Who Risked Their Lives to
Bring Medicine into the Modern Age

MAVERICKS, MIRACLES, AND MEDICINE

The Pioneers Who Risked Their Lives to
Bring Medicine into the Modern Age

JULIE M. FENSTER

The Companion to The History Channel® series
Mavericks, Miracles, and Medicine
created for the History Channel by Jeffrey Tuchman

THE HISTORY CHANNEL.

CARROLL & GRAF PUBLISHERS
NEW YORK

Dedicated to Paul M. Birchmeyer

MAVERICKS, MIRACLES, AND MEDICINE

Carroll & Graf Publishers
An Imprint of Avalon Publishing Group Inc.
161 William St., 16th Floor
New York, NY 10038

First Carroll & Graf edition 2003

Library of Congress Cataloging-in-Publication Data is available.

ISBN: 0-7867-1236-8

Interior design by Paul Paddock
Printed in the United States of America
Distributed by Publishers Group West

Contents

III.
MAGIC BULLETS

IV.
THE MIND

ILLUSTRATIONS

ACKNOWLEDGMENTS

When Susan Werbe, the Vice President of Documentary Programming for The History Channel® approached Jeff Tuchman with the idea that eventually became *Mavericks, Miracles, and Medicine* it seemed like a fortuitous match. As a documentary filmmaker for the past fifteen years, and the son of a physician for many more than that, Jeff was intrigued by the opportunity to explore the human side of medical progress. The four-part television program that he wrote and directed for the History Channel was constructed around four actual patients undergoing treatment for heart failure, epilepsy, tuberculosis, and liver disease. In each hour-long episode, Jeff traced five break-throughs that eventually led to today's methods—and miracles. He and his producer, Megan Cogswell, were very particular in making their choices. Each breakthrough they selected was the result of individual effort and, very often, sacrifice.

Jeff and his company, Documania Films, started working on the television show in 2001. It is scheduled to air in September, 2003. (I just spoke to him on the telephone and he is still at work on a few details.) For the core team collected to produce it, the show was never just another assignment—they each seemed to share the same sense of privilege and excitement surrounding medical history. Alexandria Dionne was associate producer and archivist. Darcy Bowman edited the shows. Joey Forsyte was director of photography.

Acknowledgments

I know firsthand how infectious the spirit at Documania was during production of the *Mavericks, Miracles, and Medicine* series, because Jeff called me, before I'd ever met him, and asked me to appear in the show and talk about the discovery of surgical anesthetics. I was the first interview scheduled. We taped it in November, 2001. I had a lot of fun—more fun than most people have had in the rare book room of the New York Academy of Medicine. The Academy had kindly lent the room for use as a studio.

In 2002, Will Balliett at Avalon Publishing Group, with the blessing of Carrie Trimmer at A&E Television Networks, commissioned a book to be issued concurrently with the premiere of *Mavericks, Miracles, and Medicine* on television. Joelle Delbourgo, in her capacity as a literary agent in New York, became involved in the project and suggested that I might be the author. Will's goal was that it should develop from the start as a book, rather than as a recast of the documentary. For anyone intrigued by medical history, that arrangement seemed to offer the strengths of each medium.

J.M.F.
June, 2003

INTRODUCTION

When obstetricians in Vienna ignored the newly discovered fact that poor sanitation was responsible for spreading puerperal fever from one new mother to another, the man who made the discovery, Ignaz Semmelweis, stood near a window under the maternity ward and shouted, "WASH YOUR HANDS!" He was left with no better choice.

Semmelweis was perfectly right about dirty hands, but his colleagues just thought he was crazy. He was not the only one in medical history to be both of those things at once: mostly right and a little bit crazy. If only there had been even more. Something fills the gap between the two characteristics, something that made Semmelweis grow hoarse in the hospital yard and turned many of the other medical practitioners featured in this book into desperados, too.

When Werner Forssmann thought there must be more to know about the heart than could be learned through a stethoscope, he didn't wait. It just wasn't an option. Forssmann fed a catheter inch by inch through the vein in his own arm until he thought it must have reached his heart. Then he galloped through the halls of his small hospital near Berlin to have himself X-rayed. Even today, when the use of catheters is commonplace, there are many people who think that Forssmann was out of his mind, risking himself as a subject. Lady Mary Wortley risked someone even more precious than herself: her son, at her insistence, he had live smallpox culture introduced into his veins.

Both Forssmann and Lady Wortley were proved right in time, and so was Semmelweis, long after he died. Forssmann even won a Nobel Prize, as did five other people featured in this book. By the time they reached the ceremonies in Stockholm, of course, all was forgiven and they were hailed as heroes throughout the medical world. No one wanted to remember the old days when they were just misunderstood.

But those are the old days that *Mavericks, Miracles, and Medicine* remembers. When individuals pit themselves against the medical establishment, and make it change, there is something more powerful at work than merely a good idea. Those fall by the wayside like leaves off a barrow, as anyone knows who has perused a vintage medical journal and spotted breakthroughs of a later era, lying ignored on the pages. Persistence is always important, although several of the miracles described in this book made good in a single day. Position was valuable, but not crucial. And if luck was a factor, it was very deeply concealed beneath the protocols of medicine, the most careful science of them all.

The only crucial characteristic is intent—intent so stubborn that it manages to outmatch that of the medical world itself. In a vast institution, such as medicine, stubbornness can be regarded as rightful conservatism. In a person, it may well be looked on as madness. For that reason, institutions have a thousand ways of pulling mavericks back into the herd. The people in this book tended to ignore them all, sticking resolutely to ideas that made skeptics look sage and mockers seem clever.

While it is one thing to risk life and limb, as Forssmann did, or reputation, as Semmelweis did, perhaps the highest price ever paid was time: John Gibbon devoted most of two dozen years to inventing a heart-lung machine. If it had turned out that such a thing really was impossible, as he was told innumerable times, he would never have been able to recoup the youth and high expectations he had long since poured into it.

The earliest story in *Mavericks, Miracles, and Medicine* is that of Andreas Vesalius, who lived in the 1500s and ignited interest in firsthand observation. The most recent is that of Ian Wilmut, the research biologist responsible in 1996 for cloning the sheep called Dolly. By then, of course, the science of modern medicine would have astonished anyone from its past, especially five hundred years into its past. Yet nearly all of the advances introduced against the odds by the people in this book still contribute to healing. From Roentgen's X-rays, discovered in 1895, to the kidney transplant operation developed by Murray and Merrill in 1954, old innovations are still marvels. Lady Montague would still recognize the wisdom of inoculation, which she promoted in the early 18th century. Selman Waksman would still see streptomycin, discovered in his lab in 1943, being used to treat tuberculosis. But that doesn't mean that any of them had to be discovered when they were—or ever.

The fact that blood circulates need never have been discovered. The same is true of surgical anesthetics. While the temptation is to think that they are so fundamental to medicine that their discovery was inevitable, there was much more to it than that. The mind of science before either discovery was very thoroughly trained against each. We could be waiting for the discovery of the circulation of the blood today, if not for William Harvey, nearly four hundred years ago. If that sounds absurd, it is only a greater tribute to the rare achievement that was his. He discovered the obvious, which is by far the hardest gift to give any era.

The mind of medical science is almost certainly still set in ignorance on subjects that have been waiting even longer than four hundred years to be illuminated by someone. Because medical progress is based as much on revolution as evolution, it will always require people like Harvey, more than any other factor.

Whenever something in medicine is described as being "ahead of its time," that phrase refers to one of two things. It is either a faint apology for a good idea ignored long ago or high praise for one gratefully accepted in the present. There is only one difference between the two—a maverick, someone smart enough to see another reality in medicine and crazy enough to hold onto to it, while the rest catch up.

—JULIE M. FENSTER

I

UNDERSTANDING
THE BODY

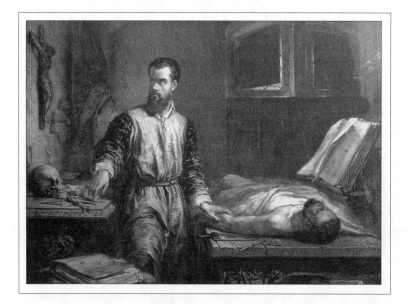

Andreas Vesalius
THE ART OF MEDICINE

B ooks produced up to the mid–1400s were precious items, found in private libraries or universities and accessible only with some sort of permission. Very few doctors owned their own books. The printing press changed that, and then changed medicine. By the mid-1500s even lowly medical students wandered around with books sticking out of their pockets and, consequently, a dialogue of ideas in their heads. The advent of printing allowed doctors even in the deepest backwoods to read texts for themselves. More than that, it allowed physicians everywhere to publish new material—the very word "new" having long been absent from the world of medical books, largely due to the slow and costly job of producing one copy at a time. Because the classics had stood the test of time, they seemed destined to continue to do so.

Printing was at the core of Western medicine's first revolution. It expanded the field and accelerated it, gave it identity and at the same time accountability. With books, the medical world was united as it never had been before—not behind any one master, but behind one philosophy of shared learning.

No one took greater advantage of that new freedom than the Belgian physician Andreas Vesalius. The most famous of his books— and probably the most famous text in all of medical history—was *De Humani Corporis Fabrica* ("Of the Structure of the Human Body"), published in 1543. It is commonly known as the *Fabrica*. Illustrated with line drawings almost as awe-inspiring as the subjects they portrayed, the *Fabrica* provided medicine with its first cogent map of the body. Just organizing such a book required a facility with anatomy that no one possessed before Vesalius's time. Actually creating it, however, took more than mere knowledge. In fact, it took more than the abilities of any one person; the *Fabrica* appeared amid a rising tide of new possibilities in many different fields that made the mid-1500s so ripe for a revolution in the world of medicine.

Andreas Vesalius would not have answered to that name on the street in Brussels when he was a boy. He was born in 1514 as André Vésale,[1] a less impressive-sounding tag, but one with its own weight in the neighborhood. His father was the personal apothecary (pharmacist) to Charles V. His grandfather was no less than personal physician to an earlier monarch, Maximilian I of Germany, and there were many other doctors farther back in the Vésal family ancestry. For a budding physician, Andreas boasted just about the best pedigree in Europe, but it was less the medical distinction of his family than its imperial connections that would stand him in good stead later.

Charles V was the Holy Roman emperor, at a time when that post was at its zenith. Officially elected by representatives of the church, the Holy Roman emperor was supposed to be the temporal leader of the Christian world, just as the pope is its spiritual leader. The underlying idea was to revive the greatness of the ancient Roman empire, though along Catholic lines. At the time Charles V was elected in 1519, the empire officially included all of Western Europe and most of the Americas, thanks to the Spanish holdings there. Through the years, none of the Holy Roman emperors had a great deal of luck in holding the flock of bickering European nations together, but Charles V proved to be an especially powerful figure. Even so, he was up against trying times. Two years before he was elected, Martin Luther had tacked his ninety-five theses to a church door. By the time Charles V was crowned king of the Catholics the Protestant Reformation was under way.

Andreas Vesalius was only four at the time, but the ferment of the

Reformation would affect his life's work, if not necessarily his religious convictions. In fact, Martin Luther was not the only person looking for some fresh grasp of the many relationships binding each individual to the universe, the state, and the church. For European intellectuals that inclination had been bubbling even within the shelter of the Roman Catholic Church, though not necessarily smack in the middle of it, for a half-century, leading to what is called the humanist movement. The main prong of humanism as it developed in the 1300s and gained momentum through to the 1500s was a voracious hunger for the knowledge of the ancient world, especially Greece and Rome.

For all the excitement surrounding humanism and the activity devoted to finding and reading ancient texts, the movement was not actually a revolution. Roland Bainton, the Reformation scholar from Yale, noted that "Catholicism and humanism were both ancient, both Roman, both universal, both Latin." There was something even more significant than that, though. "Both, too," Bainton continued, "had in common a willingness on the part of the individual to accept the consensus of the experts, a respect for authority.[2]

As Vesalius was growing up, the authority in medical matters was Galen, the Greek physician who lived from about A.D. 130 to 200. His texts had been reissued in the 1200s and gained in reputation until, in the midst of the humanist movement, they were held as irreproachable. (Before the reemergence of Galen, medical teaching had been based on Arabic texts, many of which had themselves developed on the basis of Galen's work; the most influential of the Arabian writers was Avicenna, a brilliant Persian whose writings admitted their debt to another, even earlier Greek, Aristotle.)

Like everyone else, Vesalius was taken by the scope of Galen's anatomical writings and his vivid descriptions of the body's innermost workings—knowledge that remained secret for most others. It was as though Galen could see every blade of grass on a mountaintop, where others saw only a green blur. Of course, Galen saw things because he looked, conducting countless dissections, especially of animals. But even before Vesalius had heard of Galen, he had that same inclination to see for himself, conducting dissections of small animals he found near his family's home. That made him a very unusual boy for his time; when he was older, his zeal would continue to set him apart.

As Vesalius grew into his teens, he felt constricted by the formal manner of the imperial household to which his family was attached. In 1533, the headstrong young man left to study medicine at the University of Paris. His precocity even showed in his selection of Paris, home of Francis I, the French king who was Charles V's worst enemy. For a few years, however, Vesalius was too busy with studies to worry about politics. A student who was at the medical school in Paris at around the same time made notes on a typical day:

> We were up at 4, and having said our prayer, went to 5 o'clock lecture, our huge books tucked under one arm, writing-case and candle-stick in our hands. Lectures lasted until 10. Then, after half-an-hour for correcting our notes, we went in to dinner. From one o'clock onward we attended lectures again, and at five o'clock got back to our lodgings, went through our notes and looked up references. Supper at 6 o'clock.[3]

Since the first book printed in Europe with movable type (the famous Gutenberg Bible) dated from 1456 and the first medical texts were issued in the 1470s, Vesalius and his classmates in Paris in the 1530s were very early beneficiaries of the power of printing. In the humanist tradition, most of the medical books they used or purchased were classical works, including, of course, tracts written by Galen and edited into volumes fitting the new modernity. The works of Hippocrates, Aristotle, Paul of Aëgina, Alexander of Tralles, and Aëtius were also published in the first wave of the late 1400s.

The ancient texts were treated with a kind of awe. However, a few books with more recent origins were also in circulation. One was the *Regimen Sanitatis Salernitanum* ("The Salerno Methods for Hygiene"), which had been compiled by the professors of the medical school in Salerno, Italy, in the 1100s.[4] From the time it was first printed on a press in 1490, it was something of a best-seller. By 1500, it had gone through twenty editions.

"A great many of these early printers," wrote the New York medical historian James J. Walsh, "were scholars deeply intent on the education of their generation." Book manufacturing in the first century of movable type was a lot of work and bother, with myriad steps and ample chances to ruin everything late in the process and then have to start over. "There was one very decided advantage in the difficulties of early printing," Walsh wrote. "No one felt like devoting the time and trouble and energy required for getting out a book, to say nothing for the moment of the expense, to any work that was not worth all that had to be put into it."[5]

The first relatively modern surgeon to be accorded the honor of a book in print was a Frenchman, Guy de Chauliac (c.1300–c.1370), personal surgeon to the popes at Avignon. His volume on surgery, which covered anatomy in a broad way, had been issued in hand-copied editions from the time of its completion in 1363 until it was finally printed in 1478. For surgeons, at least, de Chauliac stood on a par with the ancient writers. One can imagine Vesalius reading *Chirurgia magna* ("Great Surgical Study," or more freely, "Complete Book of Surgery") as a student in Paris—and perhaps rereading de Chauliac's extended tirade in the preface regarding the medical profession's tendency to breed generation after generation of "followers" who simply believed what was professed by others. He wished it would instead produce true pioneers, willing to study subjects for themselves and believe only what they saw with their own eyes. De Chauliac would have been dismayed to know that for three hundred years after he first wrote that admonition, the *Chirurgia magna's* followers were the most intractable of them all. Vesalius would be different, however.

At school in Paris, Vesalius grew impatient with the dissections as they were conducted for the classes. In a manner typical of medical schools of the day, the professor sat in a high chair, similar to the ones used by tennis officials today, with a small writing desk at the front. (The expression "chair," for an illustrious post at a university, is still used today.) At a dissection, down somewhere below the professor, an animal body would be lying on a table, and one or more barbers would carry out the cutting, while a proctor with a stick pointed out the detail under discussion. More often than not, the anatomy professor would simply intone the lines of Galen, adding little to what he probably regarded as the perfection contained therein.

At that juncture, Vesalius was unwavering in his respect for Galen. Nonetheless, he chafed at the stilted process of the anatomies and convinced his professors to allow him to perform the dissections himself. Rather than watch, Vesalius wanted to participate. Rather than accept descriptions of anatomy secondhand, he wanted to see. And what is more, he wanted to see a *human* body under dissection.

In France, that was very rare. In most of the northern countries, human dissections were regarded as unseemly at best. They were also considered unnecessary in view of Galen's firm direction in matters of anatomy. And finally, they were sacrilegious. The Roman Catholic Church—and most other religions in the Western tradition—regarded the body as the province of God, not as a workshop for the curious. Regardless of the religious precepts, though, there had been little curiosity about the natural world throughout the Middle Ages. Practical matters were of immediate interest, and spiritual pursuits took up most of the time remaining after that. That was an attitude that affected most aspects of life in Western Europe, not merely the lot of the physicians. Whether on practical grounds or spiritual ones, over the course of a thousand years of European history, very few people were curious about dead bodies. In fact, the stench of decay convinced the vast majority of physicians to be very devout in that regard. Human deaths were not apt to occur at the hour needed and in the vicinity of the medical school. Animal specimens could be killed just in time for a dissection.

The art of human dissection did however gain a foothold in a few of the Italian universities. The University of Bologna, which began as a law school in about 1075, gained a medical school about a hundred years later; both played a part in a murder mystery that gripped the city in February 1302. A man named Azzolino had been poisoned, or so his relatives insisted. A hearing was held immediately and the court actually ordered an autopsy—an unprecedented legal step, spurred by the progressive atmosphere surrounding the law school. A team of five doctors examined the innards carefully and deemed that poison was the cause of death.[6]

More postmortems and full dissections were conducted at Bologna and elsewhere in Italy. As to religious objections, the states loosely unified under the name of Italy may have played host to the Papal Authority, but they never caved in to it.[7] The accommodation for dissections, however it was managed, gave rise to a true modern anatomist, Mondino de' Luzzi, a professor at the University of Bologna. With the ability to study the body firsthand, he wrote a book in 1316, *The Anothomia,* entirely on the subject of anatomy. It was a good book, if not a major breakthrough. As Charles Singer explained in his survey *A Short History of Anatomy,* "Mondino is [in the *Anothomia*] yet relying almost entirely on Arabian authorities. He is really dissecting to memorize his textbook, not to enlarge knowledge, not to make discoveries. The scientific spirit has hardly awakened in Mondino. Nevertheless, he has made a great step forward."[8]

The printers of the next century certainly thought so. In 1493, Mondino's book was published with several new illustrations, in full color. Using a four-step process, the craftsmen laid down one shade at a time, using stencils. The Ketham edition (named for the illustrator) of the *Anothomia* exemplified the devotion that awaited worthy medical texts during the first century of movable type (1456–1556).

At school in Paris, Vesalius was still feeling disgruntled, even after he badgered his professors into letting him work the knives and scalpels during dissections. In appearance, Vesalius seems to have had a compact build, with wavy hair combed close to his head. In a portrait included with the *Fabrica,* he was shown as a man of dark hair and complexion, with large, searching eyes. While there is no reason to doubt the ability of the *Fabrica*'s artist to accurately portray Vesalius, biographers feel cheated by the lack of a consensus among contemporary portraits as to just exactly what Vesalius looked like.[9] On his personality, however, there was agreement.

Andreas Vesalius was a confirmed introvert, whose moods, where they were detectable, tended to be morose. In 1566, someone who knew him wrote, "*Vesalius natura taciturnus et melancholicus.*"[10]

If Vesalius was taciturn and melancholy, that didn't make him bashful. In his later writings, Vesalius could be insulting to other physicians, and presumably he was no more constrained in his dealings with colleagues and students. Yet he was universally respected. He seemed to have no use for literary correspondence of the type that engaged educated people of the 1500s, through which they discussed current events. In fact, Vesalius made very little time for letters of any kind.[11] There were those who called him a tightwad with his money; he seems to have been just as parsimonious with his time and his company. He did have a small circle of friends, though, most of whom he'd known since his youth.

Charles V chose, inconsiderately, the eve of Vesalius's graduation from medical school in early 1535 to march with an army toward Paris, hoping to settle a list of grudges he held against Francis I. Out of loyalty to his family's benefactor as well as a certain element of self-preservation, Vesalius quit both his school and the city in order to join his father in caring for Charles's soldiers. For about two years after the short war concluded, he occupied himself in editing new publications containing Galen's writing. In 1537, however, Vesalius finally did the inevitable: He moved to Italy.

For anatomists in the early 1500s, Italy was like an island where there were no limits. At twenty-two, Vesalius was offered a post as a professor of anatomy at the University of Padua. His only obligation was to conduct three or four public dissections per year, but Vesalius had every intention of overachieving in that regard.

Unfortunately, to secure the number of cadavers required, Vesalius and his students resorted to grave-robbing and other activities almost as nefarious. The problem eased quite a lot when a sympathetic magistrate who heard of Vesalius's plight coordinated criminal executions in order to suit the young professor's needs both in terms of scheduling and means of execution.[12] Vesalius drew large audiences for his dissections and was finally free to pursue his research with the passion he had long held for anatomy but had also held back. Still in his early twenties, he was ready to pull far out ahead of the pack in medicine, amid the more liberal attitudes of Italy.

Vesalius was fortunate enough to be working on the crest of three major trends surging through European culture. The advent of printing was one. The accommodation of new ideas, starting with spirituality, was the other, under the mantle of the Reformation. (Vesalius did not directly concern himself with the religious revolution, but it was all around him; his "lab partner," or fellow assistant at the University of Paris had been Michael Servetus,[13] a brilliant medical theorist who seemed to be headed toward the same conclusions about circulation that William Harvey reached a hundred years later, except that he felt compelled to express opinions about the Holy Trinity and related matters that resulted in his being hunted down and burned at the stake by the Calvinists.)

The third trend that helped Vesalius came from the world of art. Until the mid-1400s, European paintings were two-dimensional, lacking perspective and proportion. The "naturalist" artists who emerged in the late 1400s were determined to make a radical change and find ways to depict the human form more realistically. Leaders in the art community such as Verrochio, Michelangelo, Raphael, and, of course, Leonardo da Vinci were all looking outward in the scientific sense, making observations and using them to merge the natural world into their paintings or sculptures. More to the point, they were doing their own dissections in order to understand the human body. Leonardo was even planning to publish his own book of anatomical drawings, but unfortunately his collaborator died. Well-known artists of the time operated studios, or schools, where apprentices could hone their skills. One of the most respected studios was that of the Venetian painter Titian (1477-1576), a favorite of Charles V, who not only commissioned dozens of paintings from him but made him a count of the Palatinate, a knight of the Golden Spur, and a member of the royal household. Most of the time, however, Titian chose to remain a member of his own household in Venice.

In 1540, when Andreas Vesalius started work on the *Fabrica,* he turned to the Titian studio for the illustrations. He had been there before and had formed a working relationship with one of the artists, a fellow Fleming called John Stephan of Calcar—or Ioannis Stephani Calcarensis, to put him on an equal footing with Andreas Vesalius Bruxselensis. The two transplanted Belgians had produced a small book in Italy in 1538. Four years later, when John Stephen was in his late thirties and Vesalius was about twenty-seven, they started work on the *Fabrica.* Charles V, with his connection to Vesalius and his constant promotion of Titian, may well have arranged the collaboration. Indeed, in view of Vesalius's position as the son of a favorite in the imperial household, there wasn't much chance of his being turned away in Venice.

No one is certain just how Vesalius worked in creating the *Fabrica.* The only record he left was the carping he included in the preface regarding the artists—and he didn't credit any person by name. But the book's importance rested as much on the stunning illustrations as on the descriptions that accompanied them. Both elements worked together to launch the scientific method in medicine. And so the issue of the artistry is essential to the greatness of the *Fabrica.* The illustrations were probably rendered by more than one artist, but predominantly John Stephen; the most creditable authority for that fact was the artist Giorgio Vasari, who was in

Venice when the anatomical drawings were being done. In describing the studio of Titian, Vasari wrote:

> There was with him, among the others, Giovanni [John], the Fleming, who in figures both small and large was a well-praised master, and in portraits marvelous, as is seen in Naples, where he lived for a time and finally died. Also by his hand—and they do him honor for all time—were the illustrations of the anatomies, which Andreas Vesalius had carved [into woodblocks] and sent abroad with his work.[14]

The lofty reputation of such early Renaissance artists has even cast doubt on Vesalius's role in the production of the illustrations—and the book itself: Art historian William M. Ivins Jr. made a convincing argument in the 1930s that Vesalius didn't have *time* between December 1537, when he arrived in Padua, and August 1542, when he finished work on the *Fabrica,* to absorb enough information about anatomy to fill a whole book. Under the circumstances of the times, it is indeed perfectly possible that John Stephen had learned more about human anatomy in art class than Andreas Vesalius did in medical school. "As we look back over this fragmentary and frequently ambiguous story," Ivins wrote of the process, "may we not be justified in thinking that perhaps it was the more mature John Stephen . . . that was the silent, but nonetheless real, entrepreneur of those two books [the *Fabrica* and its shorter companion edition, the *Epitome*] and that Vesalius's part in their making was that of the ambitious young medical man who had been called in to provide a commentary on John Stephen's woodcuts? Such things have been known to happen . . ."[15]

Vesalius may well have been inspired by the anatomical drawings made by his countryman, John Stephen, and by other artists, including Leonardo. There was an air of inevitability about his role as author of the book, however. "Vesalius was a very characteristic product of his age," Singer wrote. "His intellectual father was the

Galenic Science that had gone before him. His mother was that fair creature, the new Art, then in the very bloom of her youth. Until these two had come together there could be no Vesalius. When these two had come together, there had to be a Vesalius."[16]

With the power of printing, moreover, there was a Vesalius for all the ages. The *Fabrica* consisted of 650 pages, organized into seven sections according to function, starting, for example, with the skeleton. The text, which seemed to have been taken from Vesalius's spoken lectures, was carefully cross-referenced, with notes in the margins making every overlapping fact as clear as possible. Even about the bones in the human body, which would seem to be more straightforward in research terms than nerves or any other soft tissue, the *Fabrica* corrected many earlier misunderstandings, including, for example, Galen's pronouncement that the jawbone was composed of two pieces. As Vesalius wrote, with the unshakable certainty of a man who had seen many an example, the jaw was one bone, not two. Galen was wrong about that and a great many other points that Vesalius was disposed and even compelled to correct.

No expense was spared in the production of the *Fabrica*. Vesalius personally transported the woodblocks along with his manuscript to Basel, Switzerland, home of Johannes Operinus, the finest printer for such a complicated job. To make the trip, he had to cross the Alps, along trails that were too narrow for a carriage or even a cart. He and the precious woodblocks went by donkey. Though Vesalius came from a wealthy family and made a good living for himself, it is not clear that he paid for the expensive printing order. John Stephen footed the bills at least initially; whether Charles V might have been a sponsor is not known, though it is plausible.

Breathtaking in every way—content, execution, and tone—the *Fabrica* was an immediate success when it was issued in 1543. For the first time, the medical world had a graphic depiction of the human body in a comprehensive and accurate volume. In 1943, a medical school challenged its students to find as many inaccuracies as they could in the illustrations for the chapter on muscles in the

Fabrica. Two students tied for first place by citing twenty-one mistakes, most of them fairly minor.[17] That would be roughly equivalent to taking a map made in 1543 of, say, all of the mountains in the world, and comparing it to the best version made with satellite imaging today, and finding only twenty-one errors. Not all of the chapters were as good as those on bones and muscles, and some betrayed a continued reliance on animal dissections, but the book was a vast improvement over anything ever taught before. More than simply setting the discipline of anatomy straight, though, the *Fabrica* served to wipe away blind worship in science, that instinct to follow the demigods of the classical era. The book fairly shone as a marvel of human ability, a commodity that had long been neglected in science.

After the publication of the *Fabrica* and its simplified companion, the *Epitome,* Andreas Vesalius abruptly withdrew from scientific research. Many profiles of him go so far as to dispense entirely with the last part of his life, as though the *Fabrica* were the butterfly and he was only the cocoon.

After a tour through Italy to receive praise for the book, Vesalius practiced medicine, though on a limited scale, tending Charles V and later his son, Phillip II of Spain. He didn't perform many public dissections, which was probably just as well. During one dissection in Spain, a bystander saw the heart twitch and spread the rumor that Vesalius had dissected a living person.

After long espousing the view that true scientists couldn't get married, Vesalius did. He and his wife later had one child, a daughter. But Vesalius couldn't seem to settle down. While his wife and child went home to Belgium, he took a tour of the Holy Land in 1564 on some moneymaking pretext. According to a man who traveled part of the way with him, Vesalius was rather strange about money, despite the fact that he was thought to have a lot of it. Rather than paying for passage home on a fine ship, he saved money by choosing a substandard tub that was overcrowded to boot. During a wretched trip across the Mediterranean, the vessel couldn't seem to make any progress against the waves and the weather. More than a month dragged by. Most of the passengers died onboard, but Vesalius vowed that he would survive to walk on land again 'possibly to get his money's worth for the fare.' Somehow, he lasted until the ship struck an island. Then he stumbled off and died on the beach.[18]

"If it be genius to be such a product of one's age," Singer wrote, "then Vesalius was a genius."[19] Andreas Vesalius leapt to take advantage of the opportunities that crossed before him, but he added something just as rare to them. There may have been other anatomists with almost as much ability, but none with his combination of humble curiosity and flinty self-confidence. That was the imprint that only he could have put on the *Fabrica,* and on a whole era of science to come. *I had a question,* he seemed to boast with his book, *and I discovered the answer.*

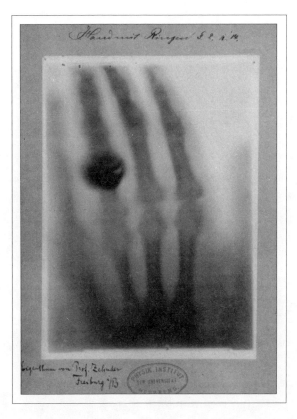

Wilhelm Roentgen
A PECULIAR LIGHT

I n modern medicine, patients are subject to more diagnostic testing than ever before, and often more than is needed according to a strict reading of the guidelines. In the case of the X-ray, though, those most likely to press for an X-ray are the patients themselves.

Practically everyone has had an X-ray, since they are used in dentistry as well as internal medicine. In either setting, the patient has little to do except sit perfectly still. In the span of about a third of a second, the X-ray exposes a piece of film with images hidden to the naked eye. The radiation inherent in the X-ray makes some people nervous, but X-ray imaging holds little danger for the patient. During the course of a year, after all, everyone on earth receives more than two chest X-rays' worth of radiation, coasting in from space.[1]

Far greater than the problem of anyone refusing an X-ray, though, is that of people demanding them. A survey of doctors in Norway showed that almost three quarters of back patients refused to accept a diagnosis until they had had an X-ray.[2] A study of back and respiratory patients in rural America concluded much the same thing: that "the perception that diagnostic radiology was needed for the best quality care was significantly related to radiology utilization."[3]

Many other diagnostic tools are available, of course, but the X-ray is the test patients have come to expect. To some degree, people feel that they understand it, and that alone is a monument to some sort of anthropological change in the human mind during the twentieth century, because when the X-ray was introduced in 1896—a kind of light that could peer into objects—no one could understand it, not even its discoverer.

Dr. Wilhelm Roentgen was the man who discovered the X-ray and connected it to a medical application. For a while, the scientific community tried doggedly to attach the great scientist's name to the mysterious phenomenon, but "Roentgen ray" does not exactly roll off the tongue—especially for those who don't know how to pronounce "Roentgen" (*rent-gen* is acceptable in English). "X-ray" is the better name, not only because Roentgen himself made it up but also because it recalls to this day his sense of mystery and awe on the night he first watched light explore beneath the surface of solid objects.

Wilhelm Roentgen was a physicist. Like Louis Pasteur, who was trained as a chemist, he came from well outside the realm of healing, yet both men helped reshape the medical world. Roentgen opened the door to radiology, Pasteur to bacteriology. In the era they launched, medicine would no longer be an isolated science. On the contrary, its rate of progress would be tied directly to its proximity to the other sciences. What medicine gained in the new epoch, more than anything else, was just what it had long needed, and would always need: fresh points of view. Deep down inside, every physician before the time of Roentgen must have yearned in the midst of a crisis to see inside a broken limb or an ailing body, but none would have wasted a moment wondering if it might be possible.

That is not to say that Roentgen was open-minded in ways that physicians were not. He certainly wasn't looking for a way to see through skin or anything else. Even after he realized that X-rays could pass through solid objects in his laboratory, he didn't instantly think to try it on human flesh. That idea came by accident. But eventually it brought him to the world of medicine, where the X-ray didn't merely extend the old parameters, it opened a frontier.

Wilhelm Roentgen was born in 1845 in northwestern Germany, where most of his ancestors had lived comfortably on plump earnings from commerce and various trades. Wilhelm's mother and maternal grandmother, however, came from the Netherlands, where his parents moved when he was three. His father made a good living as a cloth merchant, and there were high expectations for Wilhelm, an only child. The primary expectation was that he would go to college. Not many young people went to college in the 1860s, but Wilhelm's parents were absolutely fixated on the idea. In truth, he wouldn't be the first member of the family to go to college; all told, he'd be the fourth. They'd counted.

They could also, if they wanted, count all the times that their boy botched his chances. To begin with, Wilhelm was not a very good student, preferring his own methods of learning to the courses taught in high school. His way consisted of a little reading, a fair amount of hiking in the woods and a lot of sports. More tellingly, he showed an early aptitude for creating mechanical objects. Wilhelm was regarded as a precocious boy—if not a spoiled brat. He was never demonic or hard to handle, but he was allowed to grow up at his own pace and with his own private sense of discipline. After being expelled from high school over a prank (which he denied having done) and then flunking the only independent entrance exam for college (due to the grading of a vindictive teacher, so he said), he seemed to have no choice but to watch his friends leave for college. In Wilhelm Roentgen's life, the Nobel Prize was easy; getting into college was the long shot.

Through his connections, Roentgen finally arranged to go to the University of Utrecht, but not as a matriculated student. He was lucky just to be allowed to set foot on campus and audit classes. The whole idea of auditing suited Roentgen perfectly; he could concentrate on those courses that interested him most, and spend the rest of his time at the library. Within a few years, several professors who were impressed with Roentgen's powers of concentration helped to put him on track in his college career, and he eventually graduated from the University of Zürich. In 1869, he was awarded a doctorate by the same school.

Even though Roentgen tended to be shy, he was a handsome rake who dressed well and drew a lot of attention from the young ladies.[4] In Zürich, he met his future wife, Anna Ludwig, who came from a family of well-educated Germans living in exile, due to their participation in university protests. After their engagement, Anna moved to Holland to live with Wilhelm's parents so that she could become part of the family—and learn his favorite recipes. He moved to Germany to work as a research assistant to a physicist, August Kundt, who was carrying out experiments in light theory. In 1872, Roentgen married Anna. For some time afterward, he couldn't obtain a job as an instructor, solely because he had failed his college entrance exam almost ten years before. In 1874, at the age of twenty-nine, he finally left his teenage foibles behind, accepting the chance to work as an unpaid lecturer at a small college in western Germany. Under the circumstances, it was a generous offer.

Physics was an exciting field in the early 1870s, when Roentgen first entered it. Over the course of the following two decades, though, a strange fatigue settled in, as some of the old hands actually believed that everything on the subject had already been learned.[5] "The future of physics is in the fifth decimal place," said one of them,[6] referring to the fact that in the 1890s, many physicists were engaged in ever more arcane calculations on previously observed phenomena. One area in which enthusiasm had yet to wane, though, was the study of electricity, light and the dynamic between them.

Benjamin Franklin conducted the most famous of all electrical experiments in the open air of a thunderstorm in 1752, but most physicists before and after Franklin's time depended on the vacuum tube to provide an isolated environment in which they could observe electrical phenomena. To that end, one of the most important figures in German scientific circles in the mid-nineteenth century was a man without a single college degree—Heinrich Geissler, a master glassblower. He produced tubes filled with gases through which electricity was discharged by means of a coil at one end, the result being an intense color that varied, depending on the gas used. In recognition of his work, Geissler was eventually granted an honorary doctorate by the University of Bonn. A hundred years later, restaurant owners would benefit from the adaptation of Geissler tubes in neon lights, but in the meantime, the 1850s gave rise to a whole new pursuit, spectral analysis, to determine where the colors came from.

Another German, Professor Julius Plücker, refined the Geissler tube and used magnetics to tease the light into certain sections of the glass. Then he went a bit further, training the light into a concentrated emanation: a ray. Writing to the English scientist Michael Faraday of his findings, Plücker exclaimed, "By the magnet the fluorescent light is concentrated to determined places where the magnetic negative light touches the interior surface, in certain cases we get very well desined [sic] spirals of fluorescent light."[7] Plücker had constructed one of the first cathode tubes, which an independent English chemist, William Crookes, developed even further. In 1878, Crookes delivered a controversial speech at the Royal Society in London, in which he described "attraction and repulsion resulting from radiation" in cathode tubes. Crookes maintained that "radiant matter" was responsible for the negatively charged particles in cathodic rays. Even scientists who weren't convinced of the existence of radiation were drawn to the further study of cathode tubes.

In 1892, Heinrich Hertz of the University of Bonn discovered that cathode rays could penetrate a thin metal sheet, though the rays were altered and diffused on the other side. Professor Hertz had long been one of Roentgen's mentors. Philipp Lenard, a German scientist seventeen years younger than Roentgen, picked up on Hertz's work and designed a new kind of cathode tube, with an aluminum patch in the glass, through which the ray could be directed and then studied in its diffused state. Lenard's intention was to determine the quality of the ray produced: how it compared to light and the nature of its molecular composition.

Many of the best minds in physics were attracted to the study of cathode rays, believing it to be the vanguard of the field. They made up a small group, located mostly in Germany, France, and Great Britain. As a rule, they worked apart but corresponded directly with one another, remaining remarkably noncompetitive. It was a golden age for physics, one of those times when the problem in science was big enough to overshadow any problems among the scientists.

Wilhelm Roentgen had made progress in the academic world, gaining respect as a physicist and making regular contributions to the field. Known for his intensely focused concentration in the laboratory, he was amiable and active outside of work. It was a good combination for a professor intent on success in his field. Roentgen may have been bashful at times, but he had a gift for friendship and displayed a becoming humility regarding scientific pursuits. By 1888, when he was forty-three, his days as an unpaid lecturer were long behind him; that year, he was offered an enviable post as the director of the brand-new Physics Institute at the University of Würzburg, located in Bavaria, the southernmost part of Germany.

The Physics Institute was housed in a graceful building made of pale granite, overlooking its own gardens. The ground floor, with wings extending on either end, included lab space and a lecture hall.[8] The second story was the director's residence, where Wilhelm and Anna were to live very comfortably. For a physicist, it was a perfect mansion—house and lab combined, so that "working late" was nothing more than a matter of going upstairs by gaslight instead of daylight.

Roentgen experimented with each new type of tube as it was introduced, repeating the experiments of the originators and then designing new tests of his own. He used one of two adjoining lab rooms for work with cathode rays. One of his former assistants later said that the room was so crammed with tubes, coils, and other electrical components that the sheer chaos added an element of chance, which is probably necessary to any great discovery.[9]

One Friday afternoon in November 1895, Roentgen was experimenting with the effect of cathode rays on fluorescent materials—specifically, a screen that he had painted with a barium compound. Starting with a Lenard tube, he copied Lenard's own technique of enclosing it in cardboard and tin foil, in order to protect the aluminum "window" from static electricity, and also to seal light within. According to his previous experiments, the fluorescent material picked up the cathode ray from only a very short distance. Roentgen had another idea, wondering whether a Crookes tube would produce the same effect if its all-glass body were likewise covered up. He also tinkered with other aspects of the Crookes tube, increasing its horsepower, so to speak, by lowering the pressure inside the tube and increasing the amount of voltage that was sent through it.

As Roentgen fussed over the tube and its upholstery, the barium screen was sitting on the table a few feet away; he planned to bring it closer when he was ready for it. There was just one step left. He was concerned that the cardboard he'd fashioned might not fit properly, since the tube was pear-shaped. Turning off the lights in the room, he tested the covering by turning on the coil that sent electricity through the tube. The cover seemed to work; he couldn't detect any light escaping from the tube. But just as he was about to turn the current off and bring the barium screen closer for the real experiment, he noticed a green blob at the end of the table.

On closer inspection, the blob turned out to be a small section of the barium screen, set aglow by a ray from the tube. That wasn't supposed to happen. The screen was supposed to be only inches away in order for a ray to reach it. Apparently, the ray coming out of the shrouded Crookes tube could travel—it could reach all the way across the room.

Repairing upstairs for dinner, Roentgen had never been so excited in his career as a physicist. His wife, however, only thought he was in a bad mood. Admittedly, it was hard to tell: His uncontained excitement was manifested by the fact that he barely moved a muscle, except to take a bite of his food at long intervals. As he stared, he only knew that the ray hitting the screen was not a cathode ray—it couldn't have been. He understood enough about cathode rays to reach that one conclusion.

Over the following weeks, Roentgen took his meals in the lab, and instead of going upstairs to sleep as usual he worked around the clock, resting only in cat naps. His initial fascination with the invisible ray soared when he noticed a dull line running across the brightened part of the barium screen. Investigating, he realized that a wire had intervened in the path of the ray. The effect it left on the screen was not quite a shadow, though. It wasn't a dark gray mark. The line was distinctly green, if less brilliantly so than the rest of the screen. The sight of it called to Roentgen's mind an article written two years before, in 1893, by Hermann von Helmholtz.[10]

Over the course of a long career, Von Helmholtz made every other scientist of the nineteenth century look shiftless. Equally at home in math, physics, biology, and medicine, he was also a star of the lecture circuit, explaining science to the populace. Several years before his death in 1894, new research on light captured his attention, and having nothing else to do one morning, perhaps, he developed a theory. Von Helmholtz suggested that a ray of light having an extremely short wavelength would go straight through solid materials. It was a drastic suggestion, but one that stayed with Wilhelm Roentgen.

Roentgen stopped everything else he was doing to examine the wire. He realized that the ray was indeed passing through it, and not around it. Then he did a very simple but dramatic thing: He held up a piece of paper. Putting it in between the Crookes tube and the barium screen, he noticed that the ray was unhindered, continuing to activate the fluorescent paint as though the paper weren't even there. Roentgen tried a playing card, a piece of metal and a book—the ray penetrated each one, though it was at least dimmed by the book.

If Roentgen had never done anything else, the ray he discovered would have represented the biggest news of the year in the world of physics. His next act, though, made it the biggest news of the coming century in medicine.

Still exploring the effect of the ray, Roentgen held up a small lead disc. It stopped the ray entirely, leaving the screen with a shadow in its shape. Beside it, though, he saw the image of his fingers, with the bones clearly discernible. Roentgen never left any record of his thoughts at that moment. He was, however, the first person ever to peer inside a body, healthy and whole. With that, notions of the possible and impossible changed irrevocably. In Roentgen's lab room in Würzburg, life and death, no less than magic and science, were suddenly sharing secrets across a chasm—bridged by the mysterious ray.

"I had not spoken to anyone about my work," Roentgen wrote to one of his best friends, regarding his intense research in November and December. "To my wife I mentioned merely that I was doing something of which people, when they found out about it, would say, 'Roentgen seems to have gone crazy.' "[11] Anna Roentgen did find out more about it in mid-December, when she was recruited for an experiment.

Knowing that the fluorescent effect of cathode rays could be captured on photographic plates, Roentgen decided to test the new ray in the same way. Successful with inanimate objects, he wanted to try an entirely animate object, and chose Anna's hand as his first subject. While she held her hand still for fifteen minutes, the ray was projected at it—and through it—to a photographic plate. The result was a picture of the bones that made up her hand, with silhouettes where her two rings blocked the ray entirely. Nothing of the sort had ever been seen before.

A few days before New Year's Day, 1895, Roentgen wrote a report titled "On a New Kind of Ray," and sent it to his local scientific society. The essay, running to 4,000 words, held nothing back, but described the effect and exactly how it had been produced. Roentgen was frank to admit all that he didn't know about the new phenomenon, and gave it a name befitting its aura of mystery: "X ray."

The essay was restrained in tone, admirably devoid of speculation. The accompanying pictures, however, were nothing short of dynamite, showing the contents of closed boxes and, moreover, the skeletal structure of Anna Roentgen's hand.

The directors of the society recognized the importance of the discovery and scheduled "On a New Kind of Ray" for publication as soon as possible. First, however, Roentgen had to send the report to a half-dozen of his colleagues for review. "On the first of January," he recalled, "I mailed the copies and then hell broke loose! The *Vienna Presse* was the first to blow the trumpet of publicity and the others followed. In a few days I was disgusted with the business; I could not recognize my own work in the reports anymore. For me photography was the means to the end, but they made it the most important thing. Gradually, I became accustomed to the uproar, but the storm cost time; for exactly four weeks I was unable to make a single experiment."[12]

Apparently, some of Roentgen's colleagues hadn't been able to contain their excitement over the new X-rays and had passed the details, along with the pictures, along to the newspapers. The *Vienna Presse* article on January 7 was remarkably sober, considering the subject, though it did indulge in a little imagination of the type Roentgen disdained: "At the present time," the article concluded, "we wish only to call attention to the importance this discovery would have in the diagnosis of diseases and injuries of bones, provided that the process can be developed technically so that not only the human hand can be photographed but that details of other bones may be shown without the flesh."[13]

By mid-January 1896, the X-ray was world famous and so was Dr. Roentgen. In fact, there has probably never been more publicity about a single discovery, before or since. The historian George Sarton made an exact tally: "There appeared," he wrote of Roentgen's breakthrough, "within the first year of his discovery

(1896) no less than 49 books or pamphlets and 1,044 papers on Roentgen rays!"[14]

George Manes was a medical student in Würzburg in 1896. That spring, he attended a lecture by Professor Roentgen:

> When he came in, we stamped the floor enthusiastically for minutes, the customary form of applause in German universities.
>
> Roentgen, a tall, husky, good-looking Rhinelander with thick, wavy dark brown hair and a long beard, was a great scientist and an excellent experimenter whose demonstrations seldom failed. However, he was one of the shyest men I have ever met. As a matter of fact, he could not speak three words before a meeting without preparation. Therefore, confronted with our acclamation he stood dumbfounded and looked helplessly at us like a terrified child until he was composed enough to begin his scheduled lecture without any other comment.
>
> . . . A few weeks later when in his lectures he came to the appropriate section of the course, he reported his discovery in such an objective manner that anyone who did not know he was the discoverer would not have guessed it.[15]

One year after Roentgen's finding was announced, the French physicist Antoine Henri Becquerel built upon the knowledge provided by the X-ray, proving the presence of radioactivity in uranium. At his invitation, Pierre and Marie Curie took over his research and devoted all of their time to investigating radiation and radioactive materials.[16] The X-ray started a revolution in physics, launched on the recognition that not everything in the natural world could be *seen,* in the old sense of the word. Newly discovered phenomena (such as X-rays) revealed previously unknown activity (such as radiation) in the physical world—and that required new means of perception. Roentgen's rudimentary arrangement of the Crookes tube and the barium screen was one. Physicists suddenly had a world of work to do, with the X-ray as a starting point.

The revolution in the medical world was no less resounding, although it had a rockier start. Reports that X-rays could see through clothing kindled a kind of hysteria among modest people everywhere, and led to a fortune for the Londoner who rushed "X-ray-proof underwear" into stores. Other people took ghoulish delight in the new invention, giving rise to a fad for skeleton portraits. They were especially popular with couples.

Only two months after Roentgen's announcement, doctors in the United States were using X-ray equipment of their own making.[17] Medical supply houses didn't take much more time to put commercial machines on the market.

The first labs in hospitals opened in March 1896—only four months after Roentgen detected the very first X-ray. Taking clear pictures required expertise, though, and interpreting them required a whole host of new skills. As Vesalius had once pointed out, anatomy can vary from person to person on specific points; X-rays proved that, as doctors pondered unexpected features in the pictures and wondered whether they were looking at abnormalities or acceptable variances. To improve the pictures and understand them, radiology was established as a medical specialty in 1896. It didn't take long for physicians to begin experimenting with the injection of liquids that would highlight particular organs. Established surgeons were inclined to bristle when radiologists presumed to give them direction on specific cases,[18] but before long, there was no choice in the matter.

The field was becoming more complex by the week. In April 1896, Dr. Francis Williams of Boston, one of the first full-time radiologists, refined a technique for using X-rays on the lungs to find spots indicating tuberculosis, cancer, or other diseases. Williams was also the first to appreciate that the X-ray was not only a diagnostic tool but also a therapeutic one. Realizing that X-rays had the power of penetration, he used them in November to treat a breast cancer

patient, in order to alleviate her pain and possibly reverse her con-
dition. That was the beginning of the use of X-rays in treatment.
Another of the early researchers into the new technology was
Thomas Edison.

If the potential of the X-ray was immediately recognized, its
dangers were slower to emerge. Many of the early researchers
exposed themselves to radiation for hours at a stretch. Skin lesions
very often developed, along with hair loss and other temporary
symptoms, but the intrepid doctors continued on, using their own
bodies in experiments with the invisible rays. By 1897, it was generally known that extended doses of X-ray radiation were detri-
mental, a slow-acting poison retained by the body, but by then it
was too late for many of the pioneers. They were later known as the
"X-ray martyrs": Dr. John Spence, who worked with Roentgen in
1897, had to have his right arm amputated in 1916; his left hand
was sacrificed in 1930, and he died soon afterward.[19] Dr. John Hall-
Edwards, of Birmingham, England, the first person to use X-rays in
an actual medical case, was also an amputee and lived in terrible
pain most of his life. Thomas Edison's laboratory assistant, Clarence
Daily, died of radiation poisoning in 1903, after a long illness. Even
Edison was apparently affected by exposure to X-rays, suffering
damage to one eye.[20]

Wilhelm Roentgen, however, never had any after effects from his
work with X-rays, aside from the nuisance of being pelted with
every honor the civilized world could devise. For a reticent man, it
was all a tribulation. The list is too long to reiterate, though it is
notable that he received the first Nobel Prize ever awarded in
physics (1901). He accepted the compliment, but donated the prize
money to the University of Würzburg. He was also invited by the
German monarchy to add the ennobling prefix "von" to his last
name, but he declined the honor.

"The greatest and most satisfying joys the scientist can experience," Roentgen said after receiving the Nobel Prize, "are
those derived from unprejudiced research. Compared to the

inner satisfaction over a problem properly solved, any outside recognition becomes meaningless."[21]

Someone else would presumably have discovered the X-ray if Roentgen had not. The equipment was available. Interest in the subject was well established. But it is just as possible that nothing would have happened. The X-ray might easily have remained invisible, awaiting something even more unique than the right equipment: the attention of an unprejudiced researcher—with the stubbornness of a former spoiled brat.

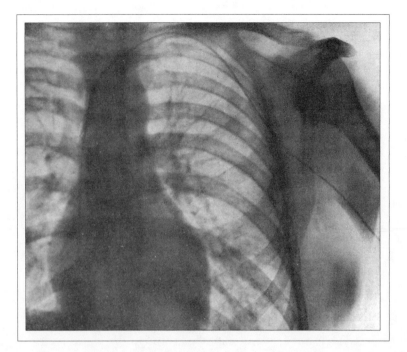

Werner Forssmann
PICTURE OF YOUTH

W hen the first vaccine for AIDS was introduced in 1987, Dr. Daniel Zagury, the French researcher behind it, inoculated ten volunteers in the nation of Zaire. Of course, no one knew what would happen; it was perfectly possible that the vaccine would trigger the actual AIDS disease. Almost immediately, the incident exploded through the world press and Zagury was condemned as a racist, experimenting on Zaireans as though they were so many "chimpanzees."

The charge struck a raw nerve, not only with people sensitive to racism, but to many who quietly suspected that in the face of any challenging medical problem, doctors were inclined to look at individuals as specimens—each one a chance for an interesting experiment. That suspicion was confirmed for the ages by the experience of Mark-Antoine Muret, a writer who lived in the 1500s. After falling unconscious during a trip to Italy, he was lying in a charity hospital, wearing the tattered but comfortable clothing that he (and many a later writer) always favored. Muret was still woozy when two doctors made their rounds in his ward, conversing in Latin in order to conceal their comments from the patients. Unbeknownst to them, Mark-Antoine Muret was one of the leading classicists of the sixteenth century. As they approached his cot, he heard one advising the other, "Do your experiment on some cheap body."[1] They then paused and looked at Muret. He immediately came to his senses and rushed out of the hospital, living to tell a story that has lasted through the ages.

Five hundred years later, the implication that Dr. Zagury was testing the AIDS vaccine on "some cheap bodies" struck just as deep. "It hurt me so much when they said I was using the Zaireans as chimpanzees," he said in 1987. "They didn't know that the first chimp was me."[2] Zagury had taken the first shot of the potentially dangerous vaccine—a fact that quelled the accusations of racism and then raised a whole new storm over the ethics of self-experimentation.

Doctors are expected to be sensitive to the suffering of others, but not to the point that that they take risks with their own bodies instead. The wavering line between those two impulses is the basis for a whole chapter of medical ethics. Undoubtedly self-experimentation is a shortcut in a field that prides itself on patience, and moreover, it is apt to be subjective, where medicine has struggled in recent times to quantify nearly all research. Worst of all, though, self-experimentation is dramatic and aggrandizing, pushing the innately threatening word "I" smack in the face of a community of medical research constructed on that more precarious word, "we."

Nonetheless, a doctor may have an idea that can't wait. In 1929, Dr. Werner Forssmann didn't wait. Leaving the whole litany of ethical questions to hang in the air, he scurried furtively through the halls of a hospital in northeastern Germany, rushing to complete an experiment on himself that would lead to a new understanding of the pulmonary system and make heart surgery possible.

Werner Forssmann was a Berliner, born in 1904 and destined to live through Germany's most wrenching era. For his first ten years, at least, he was carefree. His parents were well off and he lived comfortably, surrounded by grandparents, aunts, and uncles. Werner, an only child, was not merely raised amid an assortment of loving relatives, he was "embraced" by them, according to his daughter, in "a family that valued education above everything else."[3]

As a boy, Werner and his friends would spend free time on the

Tempelhofer Field. "Often when we were playing," Forssmann recalled, "we were able to see Fokker biplanes close at hand, and touch them ... Our games would break up in confusion when one of these little birds came in to land, and we'd go racing after it. This was about 1912 or 1913."[4]

In 1914, Germany prepared for battle with the outbreak of World War I, and Forssmann's father, a lawyer who'd made a career in the insurance business, was called up with the reserves. Like other children, Werner did his part by joining heartily in merry songs such as "Hatred of England," while lining his possessions with stickers that read "May God Punish England."[5] All of that and the rest of his world changed forever in September 1916, when he was called home from school to be told that his father had been killed on the Eastern front. Forssmann was, of course, devastated at the time, but he later realized that he missed his father in an even deeper way when he was starting his career and had no one to give him steadying advice.

By the time the war ended in 1918, neither the Forssmann family nor Germany as a whole was as wealthy as before. Of course, it is never enjoyable to be in need of money, but to be *newly* poor is to be destabilized, instilling insecurities that are hard to shake. During the 1920s, while Mrs. Forssmann took a job to support the household, Werner worked his way through the prestigious Friedrich-Wilhelm's (now Humboldt) University in Berlin. He was a good-looking young man, solidly built with shock of black hair and a wide grin. At one point, he earned money as an extra in a movie, standing around in a monocle and his father's old tuxedo. Forssmann was a fine student, but he was also known for his sense of fun and his relaxed ways. Perhaps those particular characteristics didn't help him to fit into the German medical community of the 1920s. In an atmosphere dominated by stern men, a young doctor could not be both brilliant and insouciant.

Forssmann graduated from medical school in 1928 with hopes of becoming a research physician, specializing in chemistry. To that end, he secured a residency under a famous internist—but the offer was inexplicably withdrawn at the last minute. At a time when many doctors were working for nothing in Germany's distressed economy, Forssmann was thrown into the job market. Through his mother's connections, he found a position at the Auguste-Viktoria Hospital in Eberswalde, a town about twenty miles northeast of Berlin. Forssmann was hired as a resident in surgery, though his mind was still on research on matters of internal medicine.

The head of Auguste-Viktoria was Dr. Richard Schneider, a man whom Werner Forssmann came to regard as "the confidant and counselor of my intern years."[6] Schneider was a gentleman in the best sense, who couldn't help having a good influence on a young doctor. When Forssmann took to boasting about his success in performing complicated operations, Schneider reminded him that "there's no such thing as a complicated operation, only clumsy surgeons." Though Dr. Schneider held his staff to high standards, he was as aware as anyone that Auguste-Viktoria was a backwater in the aggressively hierarchical medical community: a hospital without renown and without a speciality, which simply cared for the people in the vicinity. That was no doubt as noble a calling as there is in medicine, but one that led to nothing more impressive than the next day's work in Eberswalde. The glory of discovery was left to the famous hospitals, like the Charité Hospital in Berlin, and to its master, Ferdinand Sauerbruch, Germany's most famous doctor. In spheres such as that, Auguste-Viktoria was regarded as a mill and its doctors as mere workers.

Full of vim at the age of twenty-four, Forssmann didn't see his new hospital that way at all. "Eberswalde was paradise to me," Forssmann wrote. "Unlike Berlin, Eberswalde was as yet unspoilt by the apprehension which would soon start bearing down on us all." He continued:

Our life in the hospital was lighthearted too. Not that we interns had an easy time of it. We were always working under pressure, for there weren't many of us and we had hardly any free time. We often had to work twenty-four hours without a break. But we were young, after all, and full of life. . .

This was precisely the right climate for breeding good ideas. It was just the temperature, metaphorically speaking, to bring my reactor to its critical point. During the course of long discussions with my friend Peter Romeis, often lasting far into the night, the idea that had been vaguely hovering before me for a long time became crystal-clear. After endless debate of the pros and cons I resolved upon the action that was to decide my fate.[7]

Forssmann was haunted by a picture that he'd seen in a French medical journal, published in 1863, illustrating a doctor examining the heart of a horse. The sixty-five-year-old illustration didn't show the man listening to the action of the heart through a stethoscope, or registering the pulse with the tip of his finger. Those were the only ways to investigate the action of a beating heart in 1861, and they were still the most common ones in 1928. Instead, the doctor, Etienne Marey, had inserted a catheter (or flexible tube) into the horse's circulatory system at the jugular vein, guiding it downward until the tip, equipped with a balloon, was actually positioned inside the right ventricle. The balloon would respond to the pumping action of the ventricle and send the impulse through the catheter to a toy drum that Marey was holding near the opposite end of the tube. Marey and his colleague, Jean-Baptiste Chauveau, reported that they could hear the action of the heart with greater clarity than ever before and could even feel it, in terms of the strength of the impulses coming from the balloon. The horse didn't suffer any problems and neither did the many other animals that underwent the same procedure. The research, though never quite forgotten, was generally regarded as a mere oddity.

Forssmann, like all other surgeons and most other physicians, was continually frustrated by the fact that he could draw only a very limited impression of any human patient's heart. A small number of physicians had been motivated to look for a way to examine the beating heart, especially since one of its many secrets was so basic to the understanding of physiology: the relationship of the heart to the blood as it enters, including for example the gaseous content of the blood and its rate of flow. Those who were most curious tried to apply math and logic from afar to solve such problems, but all of the cunning in the world didn't bring them any real insight into the mysteries of the heart. "Only those who have worked through all or a part of those times can appreciate how ardently this information was sought after, and by how many devious approaches," wrote Dickinson W. Richards, a well-respected research physician at Columbia University in New York.[8]

Nine years Werner Forssmann's senior, Dr. Richards was in a position to peer as far as anyone could into the outer reaches of pulmonary research in 1928. But the fact is that he represented only a sliver of the medical community. The majority of doctors were satisfied with the parameters that kept them from fully understanding the heart, and indeed were respectful of them—the heart, in the eyes of most medical workers, was to be forever shrouded in mystery by its own sheer magnificence.

Forssmann was as impatient with that attitude as he was frustrated by risky cardiac procedures. By 1929, he began, as he put it, "to seek for a method by which access could be gained to the heart without danger, and I sought to begin *exploration of the right heart by way of the venous system.*"[9]

Thinking about the application of Etienne Marey's experiment with the horse, Forssmann realized almost immediately that entry through the jugular vein would present unnecessary risks. Instead, he theorized that he could insert a catheter into the cubital vein—which is the plump and accommodating blood vessel on the inside of the elbow. When the arm is lifted into the air, that vein provides a fairly straight path to the heart. To a man brimming with ideas, the heart catheter seemed to be assured of success. "I had no more doubts," he wrote, looking back on the summer of 1929. "Nothing remained but to try it out."[10]

Even more accurately, nothing remained except to tell the boss. The discussion did not go well. Dr. Schneider had politics to consider; he was adamant that advanced research had no place in his quiet regional hospital and that even a successful experiment of such a dangerous type would reflect very badly on his administration. Schneider knew the experiment was risky, and he disapproved of Forssmann's foolhardy intention to perform it on himself. "I know you're going to say you can do whatever you like with your own body," he told Forssmann. "But there are limits to that, too. Remember your mother. I am responsible to her for what you do. Imagine how it would be if I had to inform this lady, who's already lost her husband in the war, that her only son had died in my hospital as a result of an experiment which I had approved."[11]

Dr. Schneider not only didn't approve, he expressly forbade the experiment. All that meant to Forssmann was that he would have to go ahead on a secret basis. Like a spy, he stealthily laid the groundwork, warming up to a surgical nurse named Gerda Ditzen "like a sweet-toothed cat around the cream jug."[12] Little by little over a span of two weeks, he drew Nurse Ditzen into his plot. One day in midsummer (he did not keep track of the dates), he decided that he was ready to do it—to push a catheter through the vein to his heart. Forssmann's close friend, Peter Romeis, was present to assist, but the tension was too much for him and he insisted that Forssmann stop after the probe was only about 14 inches along. "Only" is a relative term, of course.

A week later, Forssmann was ready to have another try and bring the experiment to fruition, but in his cunning way, he made absolutely sure that nothing could go wrong, choosing to do it at one o'clock, when nearly everyone who worked at the hospital was having a nap. He also kept Romeis out of the way, but looked instead to Nurse Ditzen for help. They went to a secluded room on the second floor of the hospital.

Perhaps Forssmann did too good a job of recruiting Ditzen to his way of thinking, because as they prepared for the procedure, she insisted on being the subject. Dr. Forssmann was about to shove a rubber snake a little less than one-sixteenth of an inch in diameter toward his heart and even into his heart, if possible. Once there, it could, of course, get tangled up somehow and stop the heart from beating. That was a possibility, as far as anyone could tell in 1929. But Forssmann couldn't worry about that. He had far more dire concerns, such as mollifying Gerda Ditzen, hiding from Dr. Romeis and finishing up before nap time ended at the hospital. Agreeing that the nurse would go first, he dutifully tied her to the table, as though that were a requisite for the procedure. As it turned out, it was. He then moved behind her head, anesthetized his own arm, put iodine on her arm to keep her from getting suspicious, punctured his vein and in the space of a moment pushed the catheter down more than 25 inches. He then used his free hand to untie the nurse, telling her to call the X-ray nurse to warn her that he was on his way. When Ditzen saw the catheter hanging out of his vein, she lost her temper. But there wasn't time for that, and within an instant, the two of them were running down two flights of stairs and through the hospital corridors toward the X-ray room.

The X-rays that resulted were stunning, clearly showing Forssmann's rib cage and the shadow of his heart, with a distinct line— the catheter—curving gracefully down from the shoulder to the right ventricle. Apparently the catheter didn't cause any discomfort. Halfway through the X-ray session, Romeis came flying in, having heard somehow of what was going on, and the only way Forssmann could hold him off was by kicking him in the shins.

The first heart catheterization was a triumph in the annals of medicine, but it was also just another day at Auguste-Viktoria. And so, when Dr. Schneider heard about the experiment, he was furious. Once he was through, though, he smiled, shook Forssmann's hand, and invited him out to a restaurant to celebrate the breakthrough.

Once the smiles had faded in Eberswalde, however, the fact remained that a practicing physician, rather than an academic researcher, could not make a monumental discovery—not at a small hospital, as opposed to a teaching hospital. That was the unvarnished truth at the end of German medicine's golden age. Schneider thought it over and advised Werner Forssmann to write a paper for submission to a medical journal, but to couch the discovery only in clinical terms. He was directed to explain, as humbly as possible, that he had only made the experiment as an outgrowth of his work with patients. What he did not want to do, according to Schneider, was to imply in any way that he put himself on equal terms with established medical researchers.

To that end, Forssmann professed in the piece, which was published in October 1929, that he was interested only in using the catheter to deliver drugs directly to the heart in emergency cases. That wasn't true, but it gave the young surgeon a reason to be meddling in research. And Forssmann's background, his "excuse" for doing research, was as important to the medical community as the discovery itself—more, even.

When Forssmann's article appeared, it drew a great deal of attention worldwide and was covered in *The New York Times* on November 4.[13] That, however, was to be the high point in Forssmann's work with the heart catheter.

Dr. Schneider managed to arrange a new position for the energetic doctor as a resident in the Charité Hospital under the renowned Dr. Sauerbruch. Forssmann arrived back in Berlin with high hopes, but he almost never met the austere Sauerbruch—who was exceedingly kind to patients, but biting and cruel to the staff. That was better than the reverse, but Forssmann was unhappy in the politically charged setting, so full of intrigue and disappointed doctors. Anyway, his assigned duties made him little more than a clerk. The publication of Forsmann's article and the ensuing uproar was the last straw, and he was fired after only a month. He bounced around to other hospitals over the years, even returning for another stint at the Charité, before slowly giving up his dream of finding a place in research.

The academic setting in which all research was conducted in those days made certain demands that Forssmann could not abide. For one thing, he was never actually given a chance to conduct research, but only the chance to pay his dues, so that he might *become* a researcher someday. For a man who had already proved himself by making one bold discovery, spending years kowtowing and doing menial work was unthinkable. Werner Forssmann was a likable man, according to friends and acquaintances. But he never made himself popular in research circles.[14]

If Forssmann languished in the years after his article appeared, so did the heart probe that he pioneered. German physicians rejected it—or him, which had the same effect. In a few cities around the world, notably Buenos Aires, physicians experimented with the cardiac catheter, but with a disappointingly low level of commitment. Forssmann, for his part, couldn't pick up where he'd left off in the research. He was too busy just trying to feed himself.

While working at a hospital in the city of Mainz, Forssmann met his future wife, Elsbet, who was also a physician there. After their marriage in 1931, Elsbet continued a part-time practice in urology, the field that Forssmann eventually adopted as his specialty. Forssmann might have settled down, perhaps with a renewed effort at continuing his development of the probe, except that Germany was swirling with discontent and no one was isolated from it. While Elsbet's family flatly refused to support any aspect of Nazism, Forssmann came under the influence of a doctor at the Charité who presented the Nazi line very convincingly as a solution to the country's many economic problems. In 1932, Forssmann joined the Nazi Party. He didn't support its violent measures or its anti-Semitic campaign, but he failed to recognize that there was no way to support some aspects of Nazism without inviting all of its worst aspects as well. Elsbet didn't go along. She refused to take part in party activities, bringing official disapproval down on Werner. He shrugged it off without a care; he was still Werner Forssmann, after all, a man well used to official disapproval.

Starting in 1938, Forssmann was a full-time army surgeon, running a mobile unit in an infantry division. In fear of capture by the Russians in 1945, he surrendered to American soldiers by swimming across the Elbe River, under fire from his own side. Throughout the world's medical community, Forssmann's role in the German army would never be questioned, but he was held accountable for his early membership in the Nazi Party. Although he was eventually to be admired in the United States, he was never invited to lecture in this country,[15] because, despite all of the factors that mitigated his case, the fact remained: Werner Forssmann had been a Nazi.

During the first five years after the war, Germany was largely cut off from contact with the West. It was probably just as well. Like most of his countrymen, Forssmann was not looking outward, but only trying to find the strands of his former existence. He eventually found a position in a Bavarian town, where Elsbet also established a good practice. They made their home there with their six children.

Meanwhile, Forssmann's experiment, entirely forgotten in Germany, had found new life. In 1936, just as Forssmann was fading into the suspended reality of the Nazi era, Dickinson Richards was in New York, discussing new research possibilities with André F. Cournand, a Paris-born doctor. Cournand, a popular figure in Parisian art circles during the 1920s, offered a striking contrast to Richards, who was a quiet, rather methodical man. Nonetheless, the two men were friends and close colleagues, forming a research partnership in 1933 that lasted for more than forty years. Both had read Forssmann's 1929 article, and they decided to make it the basis of their work; throughout the late 1930s, they conducted an aggressive research program on heart catheterization.[16] When Cournand published their first results in an important 1941 article, he stated, with remarkable equanimity, that priority in the field belonged to Dr. Werner Forssmann—a total stranger in an unfriendly country.

Cournand and Richards attracted a circle of committed doctors to the nascent field of cardiac catheterization, including Dr. Eleanor Baldwin, who had a vital part in the research over the course of ten years.[17] Her sister, Dr. Janet Baldwin, pioneered the use of the catheter in saving the lives of so-called "blue babies," born with heart dysfunction and in need of speedy diagnosis and treatment.[18] Part of the contribution made by Cournand and Richards lay in revealing the potential of the cardiac catheter to a generation of physicians who then laid the groundwork that made open heart surgery possible during the 1950s. The catheter also conveyed vital information about people who had suffered a heart attack. In a very short time, the simple procedure gave new dimension to cardiology, and was directly responsible for extending the lives of millions of people.

By 1951, Dr. Forssmann was well aware of the work of Dickinson Richards and André Cournand, and was pleased by the role being played by the cardiac catheter. But he had no illusions about joining the research effort. Though he was only fifty-one, he considered that it was too late for him to catch up with the latest conclusions. One day in 1956, he was relaxing at a club near his home in Bavaria when he received an urgent message to come home. Taking a long-distance telephone call there, he learned from a friendly voice that he was a corecipient of the 1956 Nobel Prize for Medicine and Physiology. As he told a reporter a short time later, he felt like a village pastor who had suddenly been made a cardinal.[19]

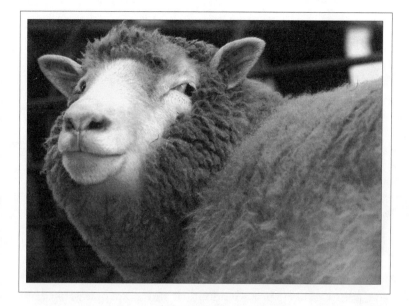

Ian Wilmut and Dolly
NEVER SAY DIE

D olly the sheep lived for six years after her birth in 1996. In doing so, she managed to outlive the craze she had started for the cloning of an adult mammal. While still quite young, she ushered in a unique moment in medical history, when a sheep looked like a poised individual and the people looked very much like sheep. For most of the first year of her grown-up life, Dolly spent her days standing alone in a Scottish meadow, surveying a herd of anxious photographers. Metaphysically, the same scene was repeated all over the world; wherever Dolly's face stared out from a magazine cover or a television feature, there was sure to be a crowd of people before it, bleating. They had only to look at a picture of the off-white ewe to express a vehement opinion on human cloning.

The phenomenon of Dolly was an important step in the science of embryology because it introduced an entirely new reproductive process—the work of a scientist in Scotland, Ian Wilmut. He announced in February 1997 that he had successfully cloned a sheep that biologically had no father, but only a mother. To anyone who heard that news, a new epoch seemed to be at hand. Very few people, however, know how to respond to news that changes the definition of what it is to be born, to live, and to die. Those are the kind of medical concepts that seem immutable, but the surprise announcement of the existence of Dolly the sheep jostled all three.

Because people are, genetically, only human, the response to

Dolly consisted of a lot of talk—some of it outraged, some panic-stricken, some funny, some skeptical, and very little of it about sheep. People wanted to know how the development would affect the human race—whether rich people would leave dozens of clones of themselves, or if a newborn Napoleon or Mozart could be struck from DNA of the old one. It was fanciful gibberish, but it translated into a way of absorbing the unbelievable, until finally, people no longer found it shocking that an animal had been cloned.

The story of Dolly began in 1986 in Ireland, where Wilmut was attending a medical conference. Over a drink at a pub, he heard that a Danish-born scientist, Dr. Steen Willadsen, had cloned a sheep from a so-called differentiated cell.[1] In a fertilized egg, which is the very first cell in the development of a mammal, the DNA is like a little director, fully prepared with the information by which the animal will develop to maturity—from one cell to a 1,000-pound Bengal tiger, for example.

By the time a mammal is roaming around, swatting flies, and looking for something to eat, all of its cells are committed to specific roles within the body. Nonetheless, the DNA within each one is still 98 percent the same as it was in the original director cell. Scientists had come to believe that in such cells, the DNA itself was "differentiated" somehow. Willadsen, working at a company in Texas, had devised a process that proved that belief to be wrong. First, he succeeded in cloning sheep from embryos that had grown as large as sixteen cells,[2] a breakthrough that gave new impetus to the field of cloning but was little noticed elsewhere. By any moral standard, Willadsen's work in cloning mammals from embryos ought to have rocked the world, just as the news about Dolly would. Earlier work by scientists, who started cloning frog embryos in 1962 (without seeing any survive to adulthood), ought to have had the same seismic effect on the perception of life—and of the scientists who were interfering with its origins. Yet while Willadsen's work was duly published in *Nature,* the same journal that would publish the first account of Dolly, it was noticed by very few people outside of the field of genetic engineering. Willadsen's cloned sheep represented a monumental advance, but they didn't become stars.

Willadsen, however, was not finished testing the limits of mammalian cloning. Developed to sixteen cells, an embryo is only barely started. The cells are still not distinctly differentiated, so Willadsen continued his work to find out what would happen when they were. While he didn't go up to a full-grown tiger and pluck an eyelash to make his point, he did clone a cow from an embryo containing 120 cells, taking one of those cells and fusing it to an egg.[3] Since he had removed the nucleus—the part of a cell that contains the DNA— from the egg, the only direction available to it had to come from the embryo cell. According to all that was known before, the egg should have ignored the direction from the newly introduced DNA, because as part of an embryo at that stage of development, the cell was indeed differentiated, ready to become a heart cell or a blood cell or a skin cell, for example. The experiment worked, and Willadsen was able to raise several calves born as clones. However, he did not pursue the research any further than that.

When Wilmut heard at the pub in Ireland that Willadsen had made the leap, creating a live cow on the basis of the DNA in a differentiated embryonic cell, he saw at once that it could lead to the cloning of adult cells.

Wilmut immediately began work on his own project. Even as he and a coworker were on the plane home from Ireland, he later said, "we were already making plans to try to get the funds to start this work."[4]

Ian Wilmut was born in Warwick, England, in 1945. His parents were schoolteachers, but he thought he might like to go into farming, so he attended the University of Nottingham with a heavy concentration of agriculture courses. He became so fascinated with embryology there that he continued his studies in the subject at Cambridge University, where he received a doctorate in 1973. Still dedicated to farming, he took a job doing research in animal breeding, improving stock through genetic methods. The independent lab he joined after graduation eventually became part of the Roslin Institute, located near Edinburgh.

For Wilmut, the creation of a clone from an adult mammal had distinct advantages over any previous possibilities, including that of a cloned embryo. In devising ways to produce the ideal farm animal for various purposes—including what is called "pharming," or the use of domesticated animals to produce drugs and even transplantable organs—it would be an advantage to see the characteristics of a fully matured adult before deciding whether or not to clone it.

The fact that Wilmut's work had a distinct agricultural purpose gave him cover from accusations of being interested in cloning out of gratuitous self-aggrandizement. However, the pursuit of profit was always present as a motivation at the Roslin Institute. Roslin was a research organization founded in 1993. Though it depended heavily on government grants, it also had close business connections to a company called PPL Therapeutics.[5] Wilmut's project may have been pure science, but he was under pressure to deliver practical results. To beg for time, he was continually trying to juggle grant applications, meetings, forms, favors, and reports. They were no easier to handle than the cells under his microscope.

Wilmut's early experiments in adult mammal cloning didn't work; the DNA would not give direction to a growing organism. Some scientists believed that by the time DNA became part of a differentiated cell, it was covered in some protective coating. A scientist at Roslin named Keith H. S. Campbell suggested a different reason. He thought that there might be only certain times in the life cycle of a cell when the DNA was activated in such a way that it could drive the growth of an entirely new being. Since DNA reaches that state when the cell it is in prepares to divide itself (the normal means of cell reproduction), Wilmut and Campbell presumed that success in adult mammal cloning was all a question of timing.

To fool the DNA into being ready whenever the recipient egg was, the Roslin scientists put the adult cell (which held the DNA) through a long process of varied immersions and very gentle handling. Most notably, they denied it nutrients at the crucial stage. Coaxed into a dormant condition, the DNA was ready to spring to action when fused with an egg. Likewise, the egg was ready to heed the directions for building a sheep. Of course, it sounded very simple, and it undoubtedly was, compared to creating a live sheep without the cooperation of DNA. In practice, the Roslin team tried 277 times to introduce a cell from an adult sheep into an egg. In most cases, nothing transpired. Sometimes the embryo, as it developed, either died or went awry. In twenty-nine cases, the embryo survived long enough to be implanted into the womb of a surrogate sheep mother but miscarried. For years, Wilmut was under pressure to abandon his project, and without strong results, funding was always tenuous. "Ian was in the wilderness," said Alan Colman, a director at PPL. "He was having a tough time justifying his existence."[6]

In 1995, Wilmut made an important breakthrough when he was able to take cells from an embryo and let them replicate in controlled conditions, a process that left him with thousands of cells containing identical DNA. He then introduced them into eggs, cleared of their nuclei, and succeeding in producing a brood of five virtually identical sheep.[7] The two survivors to live the longest, Morag and Megan, were stars of biomedical journals, as they offered the possibility of whole herds composed of identical, ideal animals. The general public, however, only barely heard about them.

Early in 1996, a cell was taken from the mammary gland of a six-year-old Finn Dorset sheep at Roslin and fused into an egg. Finally, the process worked all the way through. A baby lamb was born July 5, 1996, that was an exact replica of her real mother (who had died of natural causes a few months before). Wilmut watched the progress of lamb number 6LL3,[8] whom he called Dolly, and executives at PPL Therapeutics watched the patent process, since they had immediately filed for protection on the method used to clone Dolly.

Only a few people knew that the man-made miracle had occurred, as Dolly frolicked in the fields surrounding the Roslin Institute. She was a little large for her age, but she was no mutant who would grow and grow out of control until she sat down and flattened Edinburgh. She was just a normal little lamb.

In February 1997, as the journal *Nature* prepared to publish the first report on Dolly, a London *Observer* reporter received a tip that someone at Roslin had cloned a mammal. He investigated and broke the story on February 23, 1997. The breakthrough, he predicted then, would result in "some ethical alarm."[9] That was the understatement of the epoch.

As the story flashed around the world, Dolly's muddy paddock was transformed into a studio, from which pictures and film were broadcast showing the seven-month-old sheep from every angle. James Meek, writing in the Manchester *Guardian,* remarked on how gracefully Dolly assumed her star status. "Habituated to human attention, she is friendly and gentle," he wrote, "and convincingly feigns interest in the affairs of strangers. These are star qualities. Most stars don't have bits of dung and straw in their hair, of course. Nor do they break off in the middle of a photo shoot and, with an expression of utter serenity, pee on the grass."[10]

Wilmut called Dolly "the friendly face of science." At that juncture, it would need a friendly face. In the very first article that *The New York Times* ran on the breakthrough, a perfectly sober discussion of DNA and genetics was followed by speculation on people being cloned, even without their knowledge or permission, and also on the possibility that agencies could sell the DNA of "a great thinker, a great beauty, or great athlete."[11]

British Nobel Prize winner Joseph Rotblat was not about to license his DNA to any such agency. He came out strongly against the program at Roslin, calling genetic engineering "a threat to humankind." The British government immediately suspended funding for the project.[12] In the United States, President Clinton banned all federal funding for human clone research and instructed the National Bioethics Advisory Commission to report on the ethical and legal issues related to human cloning.[13] The Vatican condemned the practice.

After the first wave of astonishment and then horror, skepticism crept in. After all, Dolly's mother was dead, and so comparisons of tissue were not regarded as foolproof; the Roslin team could have faked it, after all, using two sets of samples from the same sheep. Wilmut's reputation in the field of biogenetics helped to contain the doubts, but they still lingered as people waited for someone to step forward and duplicate the Roslin method.[14]

Ian Wilmut was the object of intense criticism, though he was, like Dolly, a very friendly face for science. Even more upsetting for him than the accusatory rhetoric, however, were the entreaties from people hoping he would clone one of their relatives. "One inquiry was from a lady shortly to lose her father and the other was from a couple who lost their daughter in an automobile accident," Wilmut said.[15]

"It's heart-wrenching," he said on another occasion about such requests. "People say that cloning means that if a child dies, you can get that child back. You could never get that child back. It would be something different. People are not genes. They are so much more than that."[16]

Wilmut, who received 2,000 requests for interviews during the two weeks after the announcement, tried to rise to his unexpected role as ethical gatekeeper for the world of science. He cooperated with the press, but soon concluded that he was being portrayed as a monster who had unleashed the specter of cloning on an unwary world, with no care for the damage it might ultimately do.[17] The problem Wilmut could not evade was that people who didn't know much, if anything, about the subject, were convinced that if a sheep could be cloned, so could a human. It was not that simple, though.

Wilmut consistently stated his personal opposition to human cloning, and occasionally explained how distressing the thought was to him as a biologist. Hundreds of trials would have to be

undertaken, he said, and about half of the women finally impreg-
nated would miscarry. For those who carried the baby to term, the
odds weighed strongly against the child being healthy. It was a
gruesome proposition. But the public refused to focus on what
Wilmut was trying to say. "Why is it," he asked in a 1998 speech,
"that people are so slow on the uptake in understanding the consequences of this?"[18]

Consequences aside, speculation on human cloning continued.
Sports columnists named the athletes they'd like cloned and wondered, in a purely scientific vein, of course, whether a clone would
have the same desire to win as the original. Women who had no use
for men applauded the fact that with cloning, men would have no
use. Humanists decried the end of individuality in the human race.

They all spoke too soon. While Wilmut's results were eventually
repeated in mice, cows, rabbits, and other animals, the process
remained exhausting and expensive. Worst of all, the animals who
were cloned tended to be oversize and very unhealthy.[19] Dolly happened to be a fairly robust sheep, becoming a mother to six lambs
of her own (in the usual manner), though she required a heavy program of drugs to keep her healthy as she reached her sheep middle
age of four. At six, she contracted a lung infection and was eutha-
nized at Dr. Wilmut's direction. He was fond of her, but didn't want
her to suffer. Her body is now on display at Edinburgh's Royal
Museum.

Wilmut continued to rail against the idea of human cloning in
general, though he did foresee the possibility that it could be used
in cases of couples with a high risk of passing a genetic disease, such
as cystic fibrosis, to their offspring. In that case, the cells of their
jointly conceived embryo could be replicated and the gene structure corrected to eliminate the eventuality of cystic fibrosis. That
corrected cell could then be introduced into another egg, starting
the process of conception all over again and eliminating the chance
of the disease occurring.[20] That is a characteristic Wilmut called
"plasticity," meaning that the genetic composition of mammals was

not as rigid as originally thought, opening new possibilities in embryology.

What Wilmut was describing in his example, however, was not the process that produced Dolly but a variation on the one that had resulted in Morag and Megan. In fact, it was those two sheep, and not Dolly, who turned out to show the way to the future. After the first wave of adult mammal cloning proved to be a disappointment, scientists turned more and more to the embryo cloning process, which could easily be used in conjunction with genetic engineering. With the completion of the Human Genome Project, which identified the genes in human DNA, medical research gained a vast volume of new information for embryo cloning.

Wilmut ultimately abandoned adult cloning in favor of further experiments with plasticity. The man who dismissed the possibility of human cloning, however, was dismayed by the potential of genetic engineering as it might apply to human babies. With approximately the same techniques he described in the example of eliminating the gene causing cystic fibrosis, an embryo could be redesigned, as it were. If a couple wanted a baby with gills for underwater swimming, the doctors would be able to arrange it by adding a few genes from a goldfish. It was a preposterous thought, but the kind of example that Wilmut liked to cite. All of a sudden, the man who had started an epoch was himself uneasy about the future.

"Why has cloning created quite so much interest and, if you like, concern," Wilmut asked in a 2002 interview, "when I would suggest that the social concerns to arise from the Human Genome Project are actually much more serious than those that are liable to come from cloning?"[21]

II
GERM THEORY

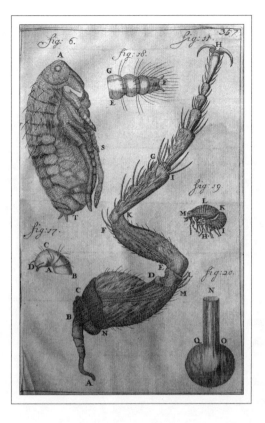

Antony van Leeuwenhoek
PERFECT FOCUS

T he Dutch artist Jan Vermeer left glimpses of ordinary life in the city of Delft, Holland: people writing letters, playing music, pouring milk; a woman in a yellow dress about to put on a pearl necklace. He seemed fascinated by the amount of life in any single, irreplaceable second, and he was drawn to that which he found in the activities of a collection of very comfortable men and women, unrushed in their pursuits and unpressured by other people. Surrounded by finery but not ostentatiousness, they reflected the atmosphere in Delft, where Vermeer had lived ever since he was born in 1632.

Antony van Leeuwenhoek was born in the same city in the same year, and inhabited the very world depicted in Vermeer's canvases. He was a burgher, a member of the upper middle class, with plenty of spare time for his interests. No evidence exists that Vermeer and Leeuwenhoek knew each other, though art historians have suggested that Leeuwenhoek may well have posed for two of Vermeer's paintings: *The Astronomer* (1668), which depicts a man looking at a globe, and *The Geographer* (1668–69), which shows the same man peering into a map.[1] Not many men in Delft studied those subjects or even owned a globe—but Leeuwenhoek did. And he had a microscope.

In fact, Leeuwenhoek (pronounced *Lay-wen-hooke*) would own more than five hundred microscopes, all of which he made himself.[2] He didn't invent the microscope, but as a hobby he mastered it as no one else ever had, revealing worlds never seen before: a metropolis in every drop of puddle water, and as to dental plaque, "all the people living in our United Netherlands," he said, "are not as many as the living animals that I carry in my own mouth this very day."[3] Making lenses far in advance of any others at the time, Leeuwenhoek discovered bacteria and was the first to see the human body on its own terms, identifying different types of cells, as well as spermatozoa.

If Leeuwenhoek had devised a way to visit outer space on overnight trips and report on the creatures on far-flung planets, he would not have made a greater impact on his times than he did in discovering the microscopic world, invisible to the human world yet coincident with it. The list of monarchs who went out of their way to stop in Delft just to visit Leeuwenhoek included Frederick the Great of Prussia, James II of England, and Grand Duke Cosimo III of Tuscany. Peter the Great, the czar of Russia, made a side trip to visit Leeuwenhoek and learned enough Dutch on the way that the two of them could converse. Leeuwenhoek was so honored by that and the fact that the czar shook his hand upon leaving that he gave Peter two microscopes. Most people who visited wanted to take home one of the magical little instruments. Very few received them.

Leeuwenhoek was no recluse, but anyone who wanted to see him and take a tour of the microscopic world had to make a trip to his house on the main canal in Delft. No one summoned Antony Leeuwenhoek or gave him orders. He was on his own by his own choice and didn't need to court favors from anyone. Asked once why he didn't write a book about microscopy, he gave several reasons. He protested that he couldn't write well enough, which wasn't quite true, and that he didn't know Latin (the common language of science), which didn't really matter. The last and most telling reason he gave for declining to publish a book was, "because I do not gladly suffer contradiction or censure from others."[4] Not many people do, but most, especially those working in an expanding field, have to accept it anyway. Not Leeuwenhoek. He remained utterly independent, straying from neither his status as an outsider nor his own front door in Delft. In an era in which science proudly rose to the status of a profession, its purest practitioner was a businessman.

Antony Leeuwenhoek lived in Delft for almost all of his ninety years. The language of the small city and its general prosperity, aloof air and commercial manners were all ingrained in him. Leeuwenhoek's father manufactured baskets designed to protected the chinaware for which the city was famous; his mother came from a brewing family and had a private income of her own. Though Antony lived for a while with an uncle, a lawyer, he doesn't seem to have had any interest in entering the professions. If he had, he certainly would have studied Latin. "I haven't been brought up to languages or arts," he once wrote, "but only to business." To that end, he graduated from a boarding school with the equivalent of a general high school education and then moved to Amsterdam to serve as an apprentice to a draper. In Holland at that time, an apprenticeship of that sort was the equivalent of a business course. Leeuwenhoek must have been a bright lad: He passed the final examinations for his three-year apprenticeship after only six weeks.

Some historians have questioned why Leeuwenhoek chose a career in drapery rather than following his family into brewing or basketry. Whatever Leeuwenhoek's reasoning at the time, drapery was the most fortuitous choice he could have made. While he was learning to inspect fabric in Amsterdam, he was handed a magnifying glass and shown how to use it in counting the number of threads in each inch of fine fabric.[5]

To enlarge a view, glass has to be very consistently curved—convex, like the outside of a ball. Because the curve has to be perfect and the glass free of pits, the early history of magnification is also the history of glass grinding. The magnifying glass, as a manufactured item and not just a lucky find in a quartz pile, has been around since about 1000 A.D., when an Arabian mathematician named Al Hasan described one in a book. Once grinding was augmented by polishing in the thirteenth century, eyeglasses were invented in short order.

Since a simple microscope is only an extraordinarily powerful magnifying glass, composed of a single lens and a holder, it too evolved with better polishing techniques and was certainly known by the late sixteenth century. In about 1590, the Dutch inventors Johannes and Zacharias Janssens built a compound microscope, probably the first one. Two lenses, one convex and one concave (curving inward, like the inside of a bowl) were arranged in opposite directions at either end of a tube one and a half feet long.[6] The thinking among scientists was, naturally, that if one lens was good, two must be better.

By the 1640s, when Leeuwenhoek was going into the drapery business, compound microscopes were popular items in scientific circles. They looked roughly like the modern microscope used in biology classes: a chimney containing the lenses was set in a vertical position, with an adjustable mirror below to reflect light. In England, Christopher Wren conducted experiments in microscopy. So did Robert Hooke, a versatile scientist three years younger than Leeuwenhoek. Hooke attended Oxford on a scholarship and although he didn't graduate, he did gain the respect of a whole circle of eminent men there, including Thomas Willis, the authority on the nervous system. Hooke would have his feuds with other scientists, notably Isaac Newton, but even as a young man, he was well established in the universe of academic science in Britain. When the Royal Society of London was chartered in 1662, Hooke was enlisted as curator of experiments. That meant that he would present demonstrations at each of the meetings, a role that guaranteed him a place at the forefront of new discoveries.

Hooke had many passions in science—perhaps too many, according to friends who admired his wandering mind but feared that it kept him from soaring in any one field. Overall, he was best known for his mechanical skill, leaving as part of his legacy an observation known as Hooke's Law, which pertains to elasticity. In about

1660, he turned to microscopy. After making his own compound microscope, he made a rigorous study of plant samples. Hooke felt sure that his advances in microscopy would bring him fame and even fortune. No one had yet written a book on the subject, so he made plans to write one. But first he surveyed the competition, asking around the Royal Society to make sure that no one else had such a book in the works. Assured that he had the whole field to himself, he put out *Micrographia* in 1665, a brisk seller that has rarely been out of print since. Though Hooke spoke Latin fluently, he chose to write his book in English, which must have contributed to its popular success, at least in Britain.

In *Micrographia,* Hooke included engravings based on his own skillful sketches, depicting sixty objects[7] such as a strand of moss, the body of a fly, and a piece of cloth. Hooke's selection of familiar objects reflected his interest as a scientist, which was the investigation of nature, just as he knew it. For example, with the microscope, Hooke could answer a question that had long perplexed him: how it was that cork could be so soft, when it looked solid. The answer was provided in his book, showing that cork is composed of air-filled chambers that he called "cells."

With that, Hooke not only put a mystery to rest, but gave biology a new word. What he didn't give it, though, was a new world. He had gone further than almost anyone else ever had with a microscope. He had learned, so he thought, just how small, *small* could be. Hooke didn't have the curiosity to press further, and he certainly didn't have the equipment. He may not have had the time, either.

Leeuwenhoek had all three. After working with a Scotsman in the Amsterdam cloth trade for a few years, he returned to Delft at the age of twenty-two in 1654 and bought a substantial house in town. The house, called Golden Head, had a shop that Leeuwenhoek opened as a drapery store. Married during his first summer at home, he and his wife, Barbara, eventually had five children. Over the years, Leeuwenhoek gained several civic titles in Delft; some, like that of town surveyor, required him to pass stringent tests, others were more honorary in character, though remunerative just the same. In the latter category was his job as Chamberlain of the Council Chamber of the Worshipful Sheriffs of Delft. It was a custodial job, but that didn't mean that he was expected to scrub out the rooms, only that he was paid to make sure that it was done. Leeuwenhoek was becoming steadily more comfortable financially, earning more while doing less. When his mother died in 1664, he inherited yet another source of income. Leeuwenhoek wasn't conspicuously rich, but he was a man of leisure in a country that valued free time almost as much as money.

Only one affirmed portrait survives of Antony Leeuwenhoek, showing a man very beautifully cloaked—he was in the business, after all. With wide-set eyes, a chunk of a nose, and a heavy upper lip, his face has a clumsy look. But then there are his hands, which are just the opposite: well-defined and almost delicate in appearance. There is nothing clumsy about his hands.

Leeuwenhoek once reflected that he was motivated by "a craving after knowledge, which I notice resides in me more than in most other men."[8] No one is quite sure when Leeuwenhoek turned his attention to microscopes. His interest probably grew out of his use of the draper's magnifier. He may also have been inspired by *Micrographia*. Another factor that is often cited pertains to his personal life. After Barbara died in 1664, he married a woman named Cornelia Swalmius, who came from a highly educated family. Little is known about her, but she must have encouraged her husband's research, since it accelerated soon after their marriage.

Oblivious to trends and fashions in science, Leeuwenhoek rejected the compound microscope. He didn't need it; the simple microscopes he made for himself were the strongest instruments in the world at the time, ranging from 40-fold to 266-fold magnification. To put that into perspective, a first-rate compound microscope in Leeuwenhoek's day provided magnification of about 42-fold.[9] As microscopy historian Brian Ford points out, the most powerful of today's laboratory microscopes are only about four times stronger than Leeuwenhoek's models of three centuries ago.[10] Leeuwenhoek's microscopes were also surprisingly small, like little booklets measuring about one inch by three inches, including the overhang of the screw that adjusted the focus. In the construction, a lens of ground glass measuring about a quarter-inch across was sandwiched between two thin metal plates. The specimen would be mounted on the end of a pin, on a glass slide or in a tube. It was then positioned using a screw that ran like a backbone down the back of the body. Leeuwenhoek usually used copper for the body of his microscopes, but occasionally chose silver or even gold. Sometimes he installed two or even three lenses, side by side on one microscope, so that he could look from one to the other and compare the images.

After Leeuwenhoek learned optical theory, he couldn't simply order the lenses he required. There was no one who could make them to his standard, so he set off by himself in the field of microscopy, first learning to grind and polish glass. His understanding of glass was so sensitive that he began to make lenses with certain specimens in mind. Very often, he left an interesting specimen in place on its own microscope, so that he could return to it as often as he liked. The result was a collection of hundreds of microscopes, each intended for its own particular purpose.[11]

A Dutch doctor named Regnier de Graaf, known for his own anatomical research, heard about Leeuwenhoek's work and investigated it for himself. He was so impressed that he was compelled to write to the vaunted Royal Society of London about "a certain very ingenious person named Leeuwenhoek." Accompanying de Graaf's letter of introduction was an essay written by Leeuwenhoek, titled: "A Specimen of Some Observations Made by a Microscope Contrived by Mr. Van Leeuwenhoek, Concerning Mould upon the Skin, Flesh, etc.; the Sting of a Bee, etc."[12] The secretary of the Royal Society, Henry Oldenburg, was intrigued enough to print the piece in the Society's *Philosophical Transactions* on May 19, 1673. With that, the door was left open.

For Leeuwenhoek, the man who didn't have any interest in writing a book, the introduction to the Royal Society provided a far more suitable—that is, *unpressured*—conduit to the scientific community. If he found something interesting and felt like writing a letter about it, he could do so. The impetus was entirely his.

Over the first few years of the new relationship, Leeuwenhoek's reports were interesting, but not far removed from Hooke's *Micrographia,* being close-up observations of everyday items. However, his microscopes were constantly improving and so, then, was his ability to observe that which had previously been unseen.

In the middle of 1675, Leeuwenhoek's work took a jump that carried the biological sciences ahead by at least one hundred years. That month, he looked at rainwater that had been left in a barrel for several days and saw minute creatures he called "animalcules," ten thousand times smaller, in his estimation, than any seen through previous microscopy. He noted the same types of animalcules in water infused with pepper berries. What Leeuwenhoek had discovered was bacteria: single-celled life forms that affect all other aspects of life on earth, including human health.

The fact that Leeuwenhoek didn't write to the Royal Society about his discovery until October 1676, more than a year later, indicates not only that he was careful in his methods, but that publication was indeed a low priority. Once his report on animalcules arrived in London, however, it became the highest possible priority for the Royal Society. A whole series of special meetings were called to debate the credibility of Leeuwenhoek's amazing letter. On April 5, 1677, a member of the Royal Society named Nehemiah Grew was asked to repeat Leeuwenhoek's experiment.

Getting the rainwater was easy. Seeing anything in it was much harder. Leeuwenhoek not only had the best microscopes in the world, but he had also devised highly specialized methods for using them. Those methods are still pondered today, since he kept them secret, just as he did his process for making microscopes. He apparently devised an array of lighting options;[13] modern microscopists believe that he developed an expertise in the sophisticated technique of backfield illumination, by which light hitting the field from just the right perspective produces a dark background, against which light-colored objects can be seen. He knew that in order to see certain microbes, weaker lenses actually gave a better view than stronger ones, if the lighting and display were properly arranged. In that respect, Leeuwenhoek had a great deal in common with Jan Vermeer, who was also an expert, and also a secretive one, in his use of special lenses and lighting effects to aid his perception of the scenes he planned to paint.

Nehemiah Grew, who was both a physician and a botanist, had extensive experience with a microscope. However, he didn't see any "animalcules" in rainwater and said so in a report to the Royal Society. Some members immediately decried that Leeuwenhoek was only a draper, after all, and could not be trusted with science. Nevertheless, he had earned the respect of a few influential people, including Thomas Henshaw, a chemist and the vice-president of the society. Henshaw, who had once tried to start a commune devoted to the study of science, was sympathetic with the position of an independent researcher.

In October, with the membership still in turmoil, the Royal Society called on microscopist Robert Hooke, who was asked to verify Leeuwenhoek's findings. Hooke and Grew worked together, but still, the rainwater looked entirely barren under their microscopes. Henshaw dourly advised them to build better microscopes.

Hooke tried a different means of display, putting the rainwater in glass tubes of various sizes, hoping to increase the visibility. On November 1, 1677, he was able to report to the Royal Society— nothing. Undeterred, the society suggested that he try pepper water, instead of rainwater.

The storm of controversy in London made Leeuwenhoek nervous. As he had warned the Royal Society early on, he didn't like to be contradicted, and normally he just turned his back on acrimony, but the battle over the animalcules was a watershed and he knew it. Though he sometimes complained that no one in Delft even remotely shared his interest in science, he gathered eleven trustworthy witnesses, including two clergymen and a notary, to look through his microscope and affirm the presence of animalcules.

The members of the Royal Society who didn't trust a draper in Delft didn't trust its clergymen, either—at least not where epoch-making science was concerned. And so the members waited for Hooke's latest results. On November 8, he reported to his fellow members that he couldn't find anything alive in pepper water. At that meeting, one member who had lost patience with the whole Leeuwenhoek affair declared that "these imaginary beings were indeed nothing else than little grains of pepper floating in the water and not animalcules."[14]

Robert Hooke voiced his agreement. He understood microscopy better than anyone else and he couldn't confirm the radical findings. Still, the society refused to lose faith in Leeuwenhoek and told him to look again. Henshaw advised him to use a stronger microscope. Despite his misgivings, Hooke obeyed.

At the next meeting, the members heard once again from Hooke. But it was a new message, as he made the announcement that ensured Leeuwenhoek's place as the father of microbiology: He had seen the animalcules, like little swimming bubbles, in a sample of pepper water. After the Royal Society confirmed Leeuwenhoek's discovery, the "new-world-of-innumerable-beings"[15] became a topic of fascination for people far outside of science. To the extent that Leeuwenhoek cared about his reputation in the outside world, he had been fortunate that the Royal Society had a man of Hooke's caliber to repeat his experiments; probably no one else in the world could have come close to catching up so fast. As to Hooke, he was fortunate as a scientist to live through the era of Leeuwenhoek's discoveries. But his own reign as the world's leading microscopist had been much shorter than he ever would have thought.

Leeuwenhoek continued his work for another forty-five years. In all, he would write 190 letters to the Royal Society (116 of which were published),[16] and twenty-seven to the French Academy of the Sciences.[17] Leeuwenhoek found "very little living animalcules, very prettily moving" by the score in his own mouth, though he was quick to add, in the interest of either science or vanity, that he was better about cleaning his teeth than most people he knew. Even more important, Leeuwenhoek provided the first description of red blood cells in 1674.

At the suggestion of a secretary of the Royal Society, Leeuwenhoek once started an investigation of seminal fluid, but it made him squeamish. "I felt averse from making further investigations and still more from describing them," he explained. However, in 1677, when a young medical student brought him a sample of semen from a man "who had lain with an unclean woman" (she had gonorrhea), Leeuwenhoek discovered the presence of a new type of animalcule. At that point, he had to discover whether it was derived from the woman's diseased state or the man's natural functioning—or the tendency of animalcules to float in through the air. For the sake of science, he put his delicacy aside, and experimented on himself, though he was adamant in his reports to make it clear that he did so "without sinfully defiling myself." Rushing with his sample "before six beats of the pulse had intervened," he was able to confirm the presence of spermatozoa. Worried about offending any members of the society, he sent his report on it in a letter separate from his other observations. However, the nature of reproduction had been a topic of bristling discussion among British scientists ever since the publication of William Harvey's 1651 book on the subject (*Exercitationes de generatione animalium*).[18] Leeuwenhoek's observations helped to move the discussion well beyond the erroneous conclusions in Harvey's book. Where Harvey was concerned, though, Leeuwenhoek did offer proof of blood circulation, since he was the first person ever to see it in action with his own eyes; he did so by devising a way to look at an eel through one of his microscopes. Concentrating on the thin membranes of the tail, he could plainly see blood moving through the capillaries.

In 1680, the Royal Society extended an offer of membership to Antony Leeuwenhoek, the amateur who had taught them so much. The nomination came from Robert Hooke.[19] Leeuwenhoek was pleased with the honor, and with the specially struck medal that came with it. If the members had been truly thoughtful, they would have inscribed it in Dutch rather than Latin, but the legend was certainly truthful, translating as: "His work was in little things, but not little in glory."

Leeuwenhoek was in his house in Delft, working on new problems in microscopy, when he fell ill at the age of ninety in 1723. After dictating two letters to the Royal Society from his bed, he died.

Leeuwenhoek had once complained about the caliber of people in Delft:

> I must say that there be few persons in the Town from whom I can get any help and among those who can come to visit me from abroad, I have just lately had one who was much rather inclined to deck himself out with my feathers [from the shop] than to offer me a helping hand.[20]

Despite his gripes, Leeuwenhoek arranged his isolation in Delft cunningly and used it to protect himself from the squabbles, stray opinions, personality clashes, and, worst of all, the conformist influences of the greater scientific community. In 1685, the Royal Society sent its acting secretary, Francis Aston, to Delft to meet the great, though mysterious, microscopist. Aston reported:

> I found him a very civil compleasant man, & doubtless of great natural Abileties; but contrary to my Expectation quite a stranger to letters, master neither of Latin French or

English or any other of the modern tongues besides his own,
which is a great hindrance to him in his reasonings uppon his
Observations, for being ignorant of all other mens thoughts,
he is wholy trusting to his own.[21]

Aston missed the point. What Leeuwenhoek showed, in his own
exaggerated example, was that carefully cultivated ignorance could
liberate a scientist.

Leeuwenhoek did not necessarily want to carry his secrets to the
grave. He bequeathed a set of twenty-six of his best microscopes to
the Royal Society. To its eternal discredit, it lost track of them in
the nineteenth century;[22] since they were made of silver and gold,
the probability is that they fell into thieving hands and were melted
down. Most of the rest were auctioned and eventually lost. Only
nine of Leeuwenhoek's microscopes exist today.

But then there are the letters. Since Antony Leeuwenhoek left
no journal of his work, his letters constitute the only record of his
researches. If young Regnier de Graaf had not taken it upon himself to inform the Royal Society about his compatriot's early
achievements, all of Leeuwenhoek's remarkable efforts might have
counted for nothing, except a gentle pastime for a remarkable
Dutch burgher.

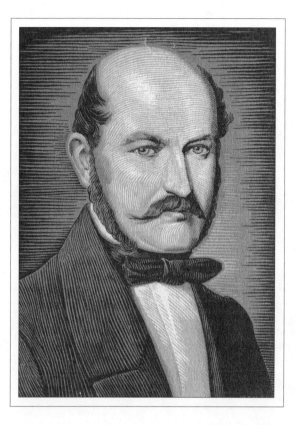

Ignaz Semmelweis
Too Much Trouble

I n the 1850s, long after Ignaz Semmelweis proved that simple
sanitation would practically eliminate deaths due to puerperal
fever, doctors and nurses were still neglecting his advice or
openly refusing to heed it. New mothers continued to die, and in
desperate frustration Dr. Semmelweis would stand outside of hospitals, as near to the maternity wards as he could get, and bellow,
"Wash your hands!"

Obstetricians had long hoped for a cure for puerperal (or
childbed) fever. In 1847, Semmelweis gave them one, and it was as
simple as scrubbing up between examinations. In clinics where he
held sway, the death rate from puerperal fever dropped from
eighteen percent to 1 percent.[1] Yet Semmelweis's methods were
mostly rejected during his lifetime, on arcane grounds of medical
philosophy or, less formally, out of sheer laziness. In 1866, a doctor
named Le Fort reported that at some hospitals in France one in
seven women died after childbirth, and one third to one half of
those deaths could be traced to puerperal fever.[2] In other words,
on a *good* day in those wards, one woman in twenty died of the
fever—that same fever that Semmelweis had learned to contain
almost two decades before. According to Le Fort's statistics for all
French maternity hospitals, one of every 29 women never left her
bed but died instead from puerperal fever. Things were no better
elsewhere. Nearly every country in the mid-nineteenth century

was devastated by hospital workers who ignored the life-and-death necessity of handwashing. Each country was disgraced by it.

And so is the United States today. When it comes to hospital infection, the jaunty air of superiority that progress gives to modern medical practitioners stops short. In 2002, a Centers for Disease Control report estimated that each year nearly 2 million patients (one out of every 20) contracts a bacterial infection while staying in American hospitals. Many are permanently paralyzed or otherwise debilitated. Ninety thousand die.[3]

Hospital sanitation is at the root all of the infections. Any sort of microbe can pose a danger as it spreads from one sick person to others. One of the most common is the enthusiastic staphylococcus aureus (staph), which can bring down an elephant, let alone an ailing hospital inmate. The main cause is the failure of hospital workers to wash their hands, making them perfect conduits for bacteria looking to roam.[4] U.S. Census Bureau statistics don't currently recognize hospital-acquired infections as a category in the official ranking for causes of death. However, according to a study by two researchers at the Medical College of Virginia, such infections would rank as high as fifth in the U.S., behind only heart disease, malignancies (cancer), cerebrovascular disease (stroke), and pneumonia and influenza.[5]

Doctors, nurses, and any other personnel with direct patient contact can make the fatal mistake and forgo handwashing, sometimes in ignorance, sometimes in haste. Even at an excellent institution such as Switzerland's University of Geneva Hospital, "the average compliance with handwashing was 48%," according to a formal study of its practices.[6] A study conducted at the Duke University Medical Center reported similar results.

Hospital workers offer an array of excuses for skipping past the sink, each of them plausible and each a veritable delight to bacteria looking for a ride to a new home. It is a reckless but sadly familiar insult to the efforts of Ignaz Semmelweis, who devoted his life to ending the spread of puerperal fever by hospital workers. For a time, he even thought he had that end in sight.

Ignaz Philipp Semmelweis was born in Budapest, where his parents were shopkeepers in a steady, middle-class neighborhood. Of German extraction, they were members of a permanent minority in Hungary, one with its own particular dialect. While that might have made them feel snug, it also left them with an accent—and gave them the status of outsiders. Ignaz, in fact, didn't speak perfect Hungarian. His German wasn't flawless either, but he was able to take up his studies in Vienna, 135 miles northwest of Budapest.

At the University of Vienna, central Europe's most prestigious school, Semmelweis flirted briefly with a legal course before gravitating toward medicine. He was apparently a bright student and did well on his exams at the medical school in 1844. His final dissertation was peculiar, though, seeming less like the work of a man of science than something an English student might have scrawled out at dawn, the night before it was due. The title was "On the Life of Plants" *(De Vita Plantarum):*

What spectacle can rejoice the heart of man more than the life of plants. Than those glorious flowers with their marvelous variety, exhaling their sweetest soft odors! Which furnish to our taste the most delicious sweetness, which nourish our body and heal it of its maladies. The spirit of plants has inspired the cohort of poets, sons of divine Apollo, who are astonished by their countless forms. Man's reason cannot bring itself to understand these phenomena on which it can shed no light but which natural philosophy adopts and respects. From all that lives, in fact, emanates the omnipotence of the divine.[7]

He must have done very well on his tests. According to contemporary accounts, Semmelweis was an amiable character. An acquaintance wrote in his diary that Semmelweis was a young man "of a happy disposition, truthful and open-minded, extremely popular with his friends and colleagues."[8] A doctor who knew him in

1847 (when he was twenty-nine), wrote that he was "somewhat above medium height, broad and strongly built, a round face with high cheek bones, high forehead, hair prematurely thin, fleshy and very dextrous hands."[9] Pictures of Semmelweis as he grew older show him with the same solid build, though his thinning hair was not to last long. After it disappeared almost completely, he made up for it as best he could, sporting a mustache at certain times and a full, bushy beard at others.

The subject that Semmelweis liked best at medical school was obstetrics. His professor in that course was far from his favorite, though. The high-handed Johannes Klein was inescapable, holding one of the most important posts in the whole field of obstetrics: director of the maternity department at the Allgemeines Kranken-haus, the General Hospital of Vienna.

In the mid-nineteenth century, Vienna was gaining status as the home of the most accomplished medical community in Europe and perhaps in the world. At the core of its reputation was the vast city hospital, endowed in the 1770s by Empress Maria Theresa. Set in spacious surroundings, the hospital was constructed of white granite around a quadrangle, each side a long block two stories high. It was a fitting monument to Maria Theresa, who was one of Austria's most effective monarchs. She was also the mother of sixteen children, and she directed that the new hospital pay special attention to the needs of expectant mothers. It did, in keeping with the modern trend of the eighteenth century, which was to establish maternity wards in hospitals.

As advances were made in obstetrics, specialists began to work out of hospitals in order to offer the best possible treatment for patients with complications. However, unless the physician insisted that a particular situation might warrant a hospital setting, wealthier women continued to give birth at home. In general, hospitals drew the tough cases, along with impecunious mothers-to-be, who had nowhere else to go. For them, a maternity hospital was a refuge and, in the case of the General Hospital of Vienna, a home. Patients could check in as early during a pregnancy as they liked and even stay on indefinitely afterward. If a patient wanted to keep her identity secret, she was directed to write her name and address on a piece of paper, which was folded up, placed on a sill over her bed, and opened only if she died. Otherwise, she got it back, still folded. In part, the hospital's generous policies were intended to discourage single mothers and others from having abortions. In addition, officials wanted to have a broad spectrum of patients on hand for the sake of students.[10]

The maternity department of the General Hospital of Vienna underwent a major expansion in 1840, making it the largest obstetric clinic in the world.[11] After the expansion, the department was separated into two divisions, a point that might seem to be of scant interest except to Viennese hospital administrators, circa 1840, but for the fact that the new organization turned the department into a very precious natural laboratory. In the First Division, patients received their daily care almost entirely from medical students—all men. In the Second Division, care came from obstetrical students, and they were all women.[12] The accommodations and the methods were identical in the two divisions. The fundamental difference was that the First Division received the unusual cases; normal deliveries were assigned in roughly equal numbers to the two divisions, which sat on either side of a wide hall.

There was one other difference. The death rate in the First Division was typically three times that of the Second. The doctors knew that the First Division operated under a mysterious curse, and so did the students and the patients. All of Vienna knew about the danger inherent to the First Division, and it was a topic of gossip in the city. Women assigned to the Second Division went quietly to the wards, but in the First Division, doctors were used to seeing scenes "in which patients, kneeling and wringing their hands, beg to be released in order to seek admission to the second division."[13] The doctor who wrote that description was Ignaz Semmelweis. He was aware along with everyone else that the difference in the two divisions rested entirely on a disparity in the prevalence of puerperal fever.

At that time, no one knew quite what caused puerperal fever, except that at some point, usually after giving birth—but sometimes before—a woman who was affected would develop a high fever with chills, followed by agonizing pain in the abdomen and head, a racing heart, loss of control over bodily functions and delirium. More than half of the women taken with the fever died,[14] although during severe epidemics, no new mother escaped with her life.

Doctors were disturbed by the specter of death hanging over what should have been joyous maternity clinics, but no valuable theory on the cause, prevention, or cure of puerperal fever took hold. Some schools taught that it was a form of typhus fever. Some implied that it had to do with the quality of the air in the wards. Some professors thought that it was connected to the marital status of the mother-to-be. One described it as a "condition due to fibrinous crases of the blood originating under the influence of a cosmic telluric character."[15] If the students were perplexed, so apparently was he.

As early as 1773, a Scottish obstetrician named Charles White suggested in a treatise that the hands of the physician just might be the cause of the fever, or at least one cause; he provided a long list of possible culprits. As far as the physician's hands were concerned, White suspected that in some cases rough treatment brought on the illness—and actually, that might have contributed, if the brutish treatment caused lacerations in tender internal tissue. However, White was closer to solving the mystery of puerperal fever when he advocated the immediate isolation of stricken women, the frequent use of antiseptic washes, and absolute cleanliness in their surroundings. In suggesting cleanliness, however, Dr. White was whistling into the wind.

Even though physicians of the eighteenth and early nineteenth centuries knew that microscopic creatures lived in all kinds of common substances, from puddles to bedsheets, they didn't think there was any reason to fear them. They didn't, in fact, fear very much in the way of organic debris. Dr. White lived in the middle of an era utterly and almost eerily oblivious to the profusion of organic matter that gurgles, spits, and sprays around an operating room. Among those many surfaces that remained spattered throughout the day, if not the year, were instruments, clothing, furniture, floors and, last but not least, doctors.

In the years around 1790, Scotland produced a cadre of very sophisticated physicians, thanks to whom Edinburgh came to be regarded as a leading center for the profession. Even so, Scotland was hit hard by puerperal fever, and one epidemic in Aberdeen added a new terror when women who were confined to their homes contracted the fever and died. Doctors were used to watching the illness spread through maternity wards, but to see it crop up seemingly out of nowhere baffled many of them. And inspired one.

Alexander Gordon, an obstetrician in Aberdeen, offered a perfectly coherent explanation of what had happened: "Every person," he wrote in 1795, "who had been with a patient in the Puerperal Fever, became charged with an atmosphere of infection, which was communicated in every pregnant woman who happened to come within its sphere."[16] Daring to suggest that doctors were carrying the disease was an incendiary idea, though, and very few people followed Gordon's suggestion that health workers wash themselves and clean their clothes between fever patients. His conclusion was basically correct, but without a specific theory as to just how the disease was carried, it failed to gain momentum, either in practice or in scientific research.

Dr. Oliver Wendell Holmes Sr., the father of the longtime Supreme Court Justice, made his own study of puerperal fever in Boston in the 1840s. He was mindful of all that had gone on in the British Isles, including the story of a heroic and ultimately successful effort to stop a puerperal epidemic in Dublin by scouring the hospital and everyone in it, and then pumping chlorine gas into one empty ward after another, just to be on the safe side. In 1843, Holmes published an article charging in no uncertain terms that it was the doctors and midwives who spread the disease. Like Gordon, he still didn't know quite how it was transmitted, but he did believe that practitioners had to change their methods.

At the time, Holmes was still a young man of thirty-three, young enough to see with perfect clarity what was wrong with his profession but not nearly old enough to hold sway over it. However, he was a unique bundle of talents, even for Boston in its flowering of the 1840s. Not only was he a professor of anatomy at Harvard Medical School, he was an able writer and humorist, well known to people who had no idea he was also a doctor. When Holmes wound himself up on the reverberating horrors of puerperal fever, he made a downright lawyerly argument, directed at the members of the obstetric profession. "Add to this," he wrote after setting down his theory of the contagion,

the undisputed fact that within the walls of the lying-in hospitals there is generated a miasm, palpable as the chlorine used to destroy it, tenacious so as in some cases almost to defy extirpation, deadly in some institutions as the plague; which has killed women in a private hospital of London so fast that they were buried two in one coffin to conceal its horrors; which enabled Tonnellé* to record two hundred and twenty-two autopsies at the Maternité of Paris, which has led Dr. Lee** to express his deliberate conviction that the loss of life occasioned by these institutions completely defeats the object of their founders; and out of this train of cumulative evidence, the multiplied groups of cases clustering about individuals, the deadly results of autopsies, the inoculation by

* Louis Tonnellé: author of *Mémoire sur les maladies des sinus veineux de la dure-mère* (Paris: 1829)
** author of "Fever, Puerperal," *London Cyclopaedia of the Practice of Medicine,* 1833

fluids from the living patient, the murderous poison of hospitals—does there not result a conclusion that laughs all sophistry to scorn, and renders all arguments an insult?[17]

The answer to Holmes was a resounding no. In the United States, his contention stirred up very little other than vitriol from the obstetric profession.[18] In a debate that lasted for years, he was attacked by doctors of many different stripes, on all kinds of grounds. In the end, though, they had experience. All he had was a theory. What he needed to even the score was a true understanding of the contagion, not just an intuition that it was out there. Hand in hand with that, he needed hard proof, which was even harder to come by. In an era long before research grants, test groups and even medical laboratories, Holmes couldn't hope to gather evidence in any meaningful statistical pattern. But Ignaz Semmelweis, taking a job as an assistant in Vienna's General Hospital, could hardly do anything else.

Statistics stared Semmelweis in the face every morning as he toured the First and Second divisions in the maternity department. For a man with a caring heart, it was a nightmare. "Only the great number of deaths was an undoubted reality," he later wrote.[19] In 1846, the year that Semmelweis took his post, puerperal fever raged as robustly as ever and was responsible for most of the overall mortality figures:

Mortality in the Twin Maternity Wards at
the General Hospital of Vienna: 1846 [20]

FIRST DIVISION			SECOND DIVISION		
Patients	Deaths	Percent	Patients	Deaths	Percent
4,010	459	11.4	3,754	105	2.7

Semmelweis made note of any and every difference between the two wards. When he realized that women gave birth in a different position in the healthier Second Division, he ordered that the same posture be adopted in the First Division. Obviously, he had no idea what caused the fever. But just as obviously, he was obsessed with it. The same could not be said for his dour boss, Dr. Klein, who took little interest in Semmelweis's panic-paced search for a way to save the women in the First Division.

One very useful aspect of the situation was that the two-sided maternity department allowed Semmelweis to eliminate most of the old theories regarding the fever: food from the same sources was served in both divisions, so the illness could not be lurking in milk, as some had suggested. By the same means, he did away with theories about the mothers' marital status, the length of labor and other factors that he found to be nearly identical between the two groups under his supervision. The differences—that was where the answer lay.

While Semmelweis continued to look for those subtle differences, the deaths continued, and for the Roman Catholic victims, a priest arrived time and again each day, carrying a bell, to deliver the last rites. "One can imagine what an impression the ominous sound of the little bell, heard frequently during the day, made upon [the other patients.] As for myself, it made me uneasy in spirit when I heard the little bell hurrying past my door; a sigh stole from my breast for the new victim, who fell before this unknown cause. This little bell was an agonizing reminder to re-investigate this unknown cause with all zeal possible."[21]

Semmelweis couldn't find any pronounced difference in the two wards, except that, as everyone could see, medical students tended patients in the First and midwifery students went on rounds in the Second. It was hard to see what difference that made; the basic care was the same. On a case-by-case basis, Semmelweis also made note of the fact that mothers who gave birth prematurely had a low incidence of the fever. Those who delivered their babies on the way to the hospital had almost none. (Vienna's poorest women, the ones who wanted to have their babies in the hospital for the sake of indefinite residence, actually took to giving birth out in a field or in an alley.[22] That way, they could honestly state that they had delivered en route to the hospital, getting a bed but not the fever that so often came with it.)

Some of the other doctors at the hospital offered vague theories to explain the pattern of fever. All of them discussed it, at least casually. But no one suffered from the tragedy and frustration of the situation as deeply as Ignaz Semmelweis. In February 1847, he was compelled to take a holiday, solely to clear his mind of the morbid images of what should have been a generally happy maternity hospital.

On returning in March, Dr. Semmelweis heard that an old friend, a male professor, had died after being nicked with a knife during an autopsy on a puerperal victim. On hearing the symptoms, Semmelweis theorized that the death must have been caused by the same disorder that caused puerperal fever. And then all of a sudden, Semmelweis knew.

"Because of the anatomical orientation of the Viennese medical school," he later explained, "professors, assistants, and students have frequent opportunities to touch cadavers. Ordinary washing with soap is not sufficient to remove all adhering cadaverous particles. This is proven by the cadaverous smell that the hands retain for a longer or shorter time. In the examination of pregnant or delivering maternity patients, the hands, contaminated with cadaverous particles, are brought into contact with the genitals of the individuals, creating the possibility of resorption [adoption of the fever into another body]. With resorption, the cadaverous particles are introduced into the vascular system of the patient."[23]

Semmelweis didn't understand bacteriology, a field of study that was still nebulous in the medical world of 1847, and so he termed the elements that transmitted the disease "cadaverous particles." Whatever the nomenclature, Ignaz Semmelweis could finally trace the spread of puerperal fever. Because physicians and medical students typically performed autopsies on victims, while midwives did not, Semmelweis could see why the First Division was singularly prone to outbreaks of the fever. Furthermore, he was well aware that medical students and professors typically went straight from performing autopsies to examining patients without so much as rinsing their hands. He had done the same thing himself for years.

In May 1847, Dr. Semmelweis issued a stark order that every medical student had to wash his hands in a disinfectant solution before entering the obstetric ward. If they scrubbed their hands with mere soap, they might remove the smudges but not the "cadaverous particles" that he regarded as essential to the fever. Disinfectant solutions, including chlorine water and chlorinated lime, had been introduced during the first decades of the nineteenth century, even before anyone fully recognized the danger posed by minute organisms. They were often used simply to combat mildew or algae. Semmelweis specified them because they eliminated the odor of death; he assumed that once the odor was gone, the particles would be, too.

In 1848, the first full year to reflect Semmelweis's regimen of handwashing, the death rate in the First Division was 1.27 percent—down from 11.4 percent for 1846, the last full year without disinfection. In human terms, the lives of approximately 310 women were spared in that one year, in a single hospital.

In only one crucial detail was Dr. Semmelweis confused. He thought that the medical community would rejoice to hear of his triumph over puerperal fever. In that, the doctor was dead wrong.

The results at the General Hospital in Vienna were either chalked up to seasonal fluctuations or simply ignored. For years and then decades, the vast majority of doctors who heard about Semmelweis's breakthrough chose to reject it. One would think that it couldn't hurt to wash the hands—that it might even be considered a relief to get other people's glop off one's own skin—but doctors of the mid-nineteenth century didn't feel that way. Many looked upon spatters and smears of bodily fluid as badges of honor, the way a gardener today takes a certain pride in hands that are caked with earth. There was an even more fundamental reason than that, though. Many doctors in the mid-eighteenth century, including some of the best, acutely resented the implication that they were responsible for disease. That was a philosophical about-face they just weren't ready to accept.

"When I was a medical student in the 1860s," a physician named Charles Johnson told the Illinois Medical Society in 1929, "Philadelphia was the medical center of the United States and the two great obstetrical lights in this country were Hugh L. Hodge of the University of Pennsylvania and Charles D. Meigs of Jefferson Medical College. Neither one of them took any stock in infection."[24]

For his part, Dr. Meigs wrote in 1851, "The contagious nature of puerperal fever, though asserted by so many of the brethren entitled to my respect for their learning and judgment and humanity, I cannot for a moment admit."[25]

Semmelweis counted on the veracity of his theory to carry it through the medical profession. To some extent, it did, as isolated obstetricians heard about his methods through correspondence or word of mouth and adopted them successfully. In Vienna, though, Semmelweis had only a few loyalists. His sense of enthusiasm, which had won him so many friends as a young man, hardened into zealousness on the subject of hand-washing and puerperal fever. He became frustrated and, at times, overly aggressive. It didn't matter: Oliver Wendell Holmes was the toast of Boston and he didn't get anywhere with his contagion theory. Semmelweis was a black sheep and fared just as badly.

For a number of reasons, Dr. Klein didn't support Semmelweis at all. One reason had to do with the internal politics of the hospital. Even more important, the two men took different sides in a shattering political struggle that broke out in Austria in 1848 over Hungary's insistence on sovereignty. Semmelweis was aligned with the cause; Dr. Klein sided with the Austrian monarchy (which ultimately prevailed). At the end of 1849, Klein replaced Semmelweis as director of the First Division; the new man immediately rescinded the order on hand-washing. One demotion after another followed for Semmelweis in Vienna. Finally, in 1850, he slunk off without even saying good-bye to his friends, to go home.

Budapest was decidedly a medical backwater at the time, hardly a showcase city from which to promote a controversial medical discovery. On the positive side, it didn't have Dr. Klein. Through the 1850s, Semmelweis lived in obscurity, practicing medicine—and making sure his colleagues scrubbed up. One of his assistants wrote a report for a Viennese medical journal on their success in stamping out the fever in their maternity clinic; the editors felt compelled to note in an afterword, "We believe that this chlorine-washing theory has long outlived its usefulness . . . . It is time we are no longer to be deceived by this theory."[26]

Germany was the only country in which Semmelweis's method found a home, as the leading obstetricians there accepted it wholeheartedly and rejoiced in its effect. Encouraged by them, and a few friends in Vienna, Semmelweis published a book in 1860 explaining the benefit of sanitation in stamping out puerperal fever. It wasn't a bad effort, readable and certainly informative, though a leader in the field later commented that if Oliver Wendell Holmes had written it, the theory might have had a better chance. Unfortunately, the book wasn't even reviled, because it was barely even noticed. And neither was Semmelweis, despite the fact that he had become more and more strident, in a desperate effort to be heard.

For a few years, Ignaz Semmelweis found respite in his family life. He and his wife, whom he married in 1857, had two daughters and a son. However, in 1865, Semmelweis's health fell apart and so, apparently, did his mind. K. Codell Carter and Barbara R. Carter suggested in a 1994 biography that Semmelweis might have been suffering from syphilis. Contracting syphilis was an occupational hazard for obstetric physicians in the nineteenth century, and Semmelweis did seem to display the late-stage symptoms of that disease: loss of judgment, insomnia, and progressive paralysis, among others. However, modern pathologists have also suggested that he had Alzheimer's disease, presenile dementia.[27]

Semmelweis's family lost patience with him, acting as though they wished he were dead. They had him commited to an insane asylum, where he didn't even last two weeks. He was beaten savagely, a factor that contributed to his death on August 13, 1865.

Two years later, Joseph Lister told the world that unclean surfaces have germs and that germs can be lethal in surgery—including obstetrics. Lister was convincing, but it was Louis Pasteur who, in 1879, finally provided the missing piece of Semmelweis's argument, identifying the actual bacterial organisms (streptococci) that cause most cases of puerperal fever. The profession was finally convinced, and practitioners adopted Semmelweis's methods. By the end of the century, puerperal fever was no longer a scourge: a rough estimate put the number of deaths at .002 percent of all women giving birth in Europe and the U.S. from 1880 to 1900. The figure continued to drop from there. Puerperal fever had only one last outpost: the illegal abortion mill, as 40 percent of all those who died of the fever did so after undergoing a procedure at an unregulated venue.[28]

With the change of attitude, the memory of Ignaz Semmelweis was resurrected and he was regarded as a hero, especially in his native Hungary. Today, there are hospitals, museums, libraries, statues, and a major medical school in Budapest dedicated to his achievement. Even Vienna, once so scornful, is now proud to count Semmelweis as a part of its history. In his own eyes, he was only trying to save new mothers from death. In a broader sense, though, he was telling a world of physicians that they didn't only cure illness, they might also cause it; they didn't only save lives, they could take them. He was right. But that didn't make him the right man to say it.

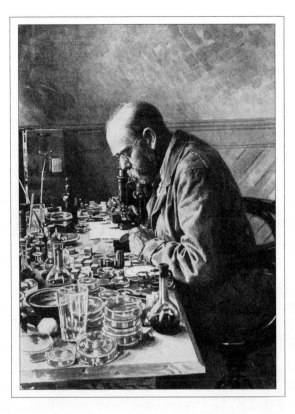

Robert Koch
PUBLIC ENEMY

O
n March 24, 1882, about a dozen people were expected for an evening lecture at the Berlin Physiological Society.[1] Nearly one hundred showed up, including some of Germany's most eminent scientists and physicians. The first seventy-four found seats in the society's small reading room, the rest stood in the back or along the sides, where tables were set up for demonstrations after the talk. For all the excitement in the air, though, very few of the people in attendance could say precisely why they were there. The announced topic was "On Tuberculosis," a vague title in an era when TB was rampant. No other information about the subject of the lecture had even been released.

The speaker was Robert Koch, a physician who was fairly new to Berlin. Though he wasn't a star of the magnitude of Berlin's own Rudolf Virchow or Paris's Louis Pasteur, he had already proven himself with innovative techniques in bacteriology. He had also isolated the first microorganism connected to a disease, *Bacillus anthracis,* the cause of anthrax. If Koch (pronounced "coke") had something to say about tuberculosis, it was bound to be new. And that is why there were no empty seats at the Physiological Society.

By the end of that two-hour speech, Koch would be recognized as the most important man in the history of tuberculosis.[2] The *British Medical Journal* would one day rank Koch among the four greatest figures in the modern history of medicine, along with William Harvey, Andreas Vesalius, and the eighteenth-century

British obstetrician William Hunter.[3] It isn't often that a whole life in science is made in a single evening. Koch, after all, had an illustrious career after the speech. But it would be just as accurate to say that he had an illustrious career because of it.

At times, Koch was afraid that he was boring his audience, since there was no sound at all from the seats. He needn't have worried. Those who were lucky enough to be present were rapt by Koch's presentation, as though he were just back from the future and was showing slides of what he'd seen. That was the view he was giving his audience in relation to bacteriology. The soft-spoken doctor not only described for the first time the organism that caused TB, he set standards for bacteriological research that are still fundamental to the science today, as are many of the specific techniques he described. Koch started the talk by justifying the subject of his research . . .

"If the number of victims which a disease claims is the measure of its significance," Koch said, "then all diseases, particularly the most dreaded infectious diseases, such as bubonic plague, Asiatic cholera, etc., must rank far behind tuberculosis. Statistics teach that one-seventh of all human beings die of tuberculosis and that, if one considers only the productive middle-age groups, tuberculosis carries away one-third and often more of these."[4] Most of the people in attendance knew the truth of those statistics firsthand, and also knew, as Koch said next, that efforts to find the microorganism responsible for those deaths had failed. In fact, many people in medicine were still questioning whether the cause was a microorganism. The old-fashioned name for tuberculosis was "consumption," which indicated everything that was certain about the etiology of the disease: the body was consumed—by something, though no one knew quite what. Believing that the cause was parasitic, Koch admitted that he had started his search of cultures taken from known victims by trying all of the usual methods of staining, without success.

"But by reason of several incidental observations I was prompted to abandon these methods," Koch said. A "virus," as he called it, had to be lurking in tubercular tissue; the problem was finding some chemical means of coaxing it into view. Through experiment and his own remarkable intuition where microbes were concerned, he found another means to drag the tuberculosis bug out of the morass. He explained the process in his speech: first drying a sample; soaking it in a special alcohol solution, for which he gave a recipe; rinsing it and treating it with a brown stain called vesuvin.

"The color contrast between the brown-stained tissue and the blue-tubercle bacilli is so striking," Koch reflected only a few minutes into his speech, "that the latter, which are frequently present only in very small numbers, are nevertheless seen and identified with the greatest certainty." He described the sight of the bacilli very succinctly, yet that image, which may have become familiar and old hat to him, was nothing less than astonishing to all others. *The tubercle bacilli . . . are nevertheless seen and identified with the greatest certainty.* Those in the audience must have been repeating those words in their minds, but Koch went right on, describing humankind's worst enemy. "They are rod-shaped," Koch said of the bacilli. "They are very thin and one-fourth to one-half as long as the diameter of a red blood corpuscle, although they may sometimes reach a greater length."

Koch then went on to tell the people in the audience about the different strains of tuberculosis bacilli, at different stages of development and within various types of tissue. He commented on the low chance of contracting tuberculosis through an open wound and pointed out that the bacteria has to be taken into tissue in which it can propagate. The outer layers of the skin won't do. Even in the lungs, certain conditions have to prevail before the bacillus takes. "It would be hardly understandable otherwise," Koch wrote, "that tuberculosis is not much more frequent than it really is, since practically everybody, particularly in densely populated places, comes more or less in contact with tuberculosis." In one of the few instances of speculation in the whole article, a masterpiece of observational science, he suggested a few of the special conditions that allow the bacilli to infect a person.

If Koch's talk had ended with that point, it would have carried the same immediate impact, making headlines all over the world and creating excitement with anyone remotely concerned with public health. However, Koch continued, in what might be considered part two of his lecture:

> If we ask further what significance belongs to the results gained in this study of tuberculosis it must be considered a gain for science that it has been possible for the first time to establish the complete proof of the parasitic nature of a human infectious disease, and this of the most important one . . . It may be expected that the elucidation of the aetiology of tuberculosis will provide new viewpoints for the study of other infectious diseases, and that the research methods which have stood the test in the investigation of the aetiology of tuberculosis will be of advantage for the work in other infectious diseases.[5]

Koch went on to describe the laboratory philosophies that would gauge the worth of new research, if scientists were to attempt—as he correctly anticipated they would—to find the microbe to blame for each of hundreds of infectious diseases.

When Koch finished speaking, he was greeted with total silence. On that night, it was a greater compliment than any standing ovation. "Everybody who attended the lecture was deeply affected," wrote Paul Ehrlich, who was there, "and I have to say that this evening has remained in my memory as my greatest scientific occasion."[6] Word of the lecture spread, even before the text of it was rushed into print two weeks later. "I always remember," wrote another scientist, speaking of Kaiser Wilhelm I, "the words of our good, old Emperor, who asked after the gala performance . . . Do you know now, how to fight this enemy?"[7]

Robert Koch was an immediate celebrity, hailed around the world as the man who had cornered that "enemy." Like the scientists in the audience at the Physiology Society, people everywhere couldn't help wondering where Koch had been. And more than that, where he was going.

Koch was born in 1843 in Clausthal, a small town in the Harz Mountain region of central Germany, where his father was a mining engineer. There were thirteen children in the Koch family, eleven of whom survived to adulthood, but Robert, the third eldest, was his mother's favorite, or so it was later said. He was a bright boy and enthusiastic about his many hobbies, ranging from collecting caterpillars to playing the zither to using a camera.[8] Although he was not a remarkable student, his parents found the money to send him to Göttingen University, where he studied for his medical degree. Influenced by an encouraging faculty, Koch developed a deep passion for research. He had the cool objectivity for it, but he was also at the mercy of his emotions, which could be overwhelming. After he received his medical degree, he decided that he wanted to marry a hometown girl named Emmy Fraatz. She accepted his proposal— but only on the condition that he would become a country doctor. The odds of Koch's becoming Germany's greatest research scientist, never very promising, seemed at that point to sink out of sight.

For a half-dozen years during the late 1860s, the couple moved frequently, as Koch found it hard to obtain a secure position. They finally found a home in the town of Wollstein (Wolsztyn), in what is now Poland, where Koch worked for the state as a medical officer while building his own practice. Financially, they were comfortable for the first time, which allowed Koch to indulge in his interest in photography. He also set up a rudimentary laboratory so that he could dabble in medical research on the same basis. As his birthday approached in 1871, Emmy decided to splurge on a gift: either a carriage or a microscope.[9] The carriage would make his life easier on house calls. The microscope was more of a hobby item. Both were expensive. Consulting with her husband, she finally decided.

At twenty-eight, Robert Koch had to ride everywhere on horse-back, but at least he had his own microscope. Emmy's timing was propitious. The debate that heated discussions among doctors and biologists in the 1870s concerned the origin of contagious disease. No one really knew the answer. Louis Pasteur had suggested that the propagation of certain bacteria within the body might cause infection. In 1865, Joseph Lister proved conclusively that bacteria was the cause of infection in open wounds. Those developments pointed to the possibility that bacteria was also responsible for disease. Papers on the topic were presented and refuted in the ebb and flow of conjecture, but no one was certain how disease was transmitted.

In 1873, armed with a new and more powerful microscope, Koch entered the fray, though no one in the scientific world would have known it, unless for some reason they followed developments in Wollstein avidly. Koch focused his attention on anthrax, a deadly bacteria that was passed from farm animals to humans, sometimes in hides or entrails. After diligent experimentation, he found a combination of stains that enabled him to see the bacilli clearly. At the time, he didn't know if the rodlike organisms were even alive, as the term was understood, but he had been taught by Prof. Jacob Henle at Göttingen University that a contagious disease would have to be caused by a "parasite" that could reproduce itself. Koch learned to cultivate the deadly anthrax bacteria and introduce it into the blood of rabbits, where it did indeed reproduce, according to his research. He refined his methods so that he could connect the bacilli to anthrax and then the reproduction of the bacilli to the spread of the disease. From the first, Koch recognized that bacterial research is not a matter of one interesting observation or discovery; it has to be part of a construction of observations and tests in order to allow for a definite conclusion. His hermetic existence in Wollstein and his utter lack of a reputation in the sciences probably made him feel defensive; knowing that no one would give him the benefit of the doubt regarding his conclusions, he made them bulletproof.

Koch's system consisted of four steps, after isolating a promising microbe: The first was confirming that the organism was found in all animals with the disease, but none without it; the second was growing it as a culture in isolation from a host; the third was establishing that the organism caused the disease when inoculated into an otherwise healthy animal; and the last was making sure that it could then be drawn from that animal and reisolated as a culture. In the case of anthrax, he completed that process after about three years of research.

In 1876, Koch wrote a letter to a well-known bacteriologist, Ferdinand Cohn, in the city of Breslau and asked if he would review the findings. "I had been receiving such communications from dilettantes, regarding alleged discoveries," Cohn later wrote. "I anticipated little of value from this request from a completely unknown physician from a rural Polish town. . . . Within the first hour, I recognized that he was the unsurpassed master of scientific research."[10]

For the first time in history, a disease had been traced directly to a microscopic organism. Koch immediately wrote an article about his anthrax discovery. It was extremely well received, yet he remained in his little home laboratory in Wollstein. When he wasn't seeing patients, giving smallpox vaccinations, or filing death certificates, he was home in his lab laying the groundwork for the study of bacteriology.

Koch investigated ways to make photographs of the images he saw through his microscope, pioneering visualization of results as an accepted form of evidence. In fact, he constantly experimented with new means of looking at microscopic organisms. He was still on the defensive, intent on finding better ways to generate proof of his findings—if not because of his humble background, then because of the many scientists who were still unconvinced of the value of bacteriology in medicine. He was determined not to offend them. In discussing objections to germ theory in his first book, published in 1880, he admitted "that the frequent discovery of microorganisms in traumatic infective diseases and the experimental investigations made in connection with them render the parasitic nature of these diseases probable, but that a thoroughly satisfactory proof has not yet been furnished."

A little later, Koch wrote a sentence that probably reflected the conceit that motivated him as he toiled away in Wollstein: "I have unremittingly attempted to improve the means for the discovery of pathogenic bacteria in animal tissue, because I could not get rid of the idea that the doubtful results of investigations with regard to the parasites of infective diseases might have their foundation in the incompleteness of the methods used."[11]

With Emmy serving as his assistant, he isolated staphylococcus and streptococcus in 1878. It seemed absurd to Professor Cohn that the world's finest bacteriologist was working in a home lab in a farm town, but efforts to secure a suitable university position for Koch were unsuccessful. In 1880, Koch finally made the transition to a full-time lab position, moving to Berlin to head his own team at the government's Imperial Health Office. He was thirty-seven. Koch had worked alone in bacteriology for eight years, but in Berlin, he became a colonel overseeing a cadre of researchers. And he was a good leader. In 1881, the team turned its attention to the search for a bacterial cause for tuberculosis.

Tuberculosis had other names, including phthisis, which means "wasting" in Greek.[12] The best theory held that the disease was caused by "bad air," referring to polluted cities or stuffy interiors. TB struck people of all ages, but young and middle-aged adults were the most common victims. It especially preyed on those weakened by some other ailment, or by overwork, a poor diet, general fatigue, and even tension. It often started as a cough, which eventually brought up blood. It didn't always start in the lungs, though, sometimes attacking the bones, spleen, or heart first. Wherever it spread in the body, it caused the formation of pus-filled nodes, called tubercles.

Many patients—especially those in good overall health—contracted TB for a short time without even knowing it. Some people had mild cases, in which the tubercles calcified and left only scar tissue. For others, TB very often resulted in a long, slow death. Loss of appetite and low energy were the usual symptoms; a ghostly pale and emaciated appearance was typical. As the disease progressed, it caused tremendous pain in the chest and insomnia. Over the years, a person could try to go about normal activities, despite the specter of coughing fits and fatigue. Because of the way victims were slowly ushered out of life, TB was a state of transition, even more than a malady. Another name for it was "white death."

St. Francis of Assisi died of TB, as did John Keats, Elizabeth Barrett Browning, Henry David Thoreau, Emily Brönte and several of her siblings, Anton Chekhov and Frederic Chopin. One reason that the nineteenth century is regarded as the "Romantic Era" in the arts is that the air of resignation associated with TB was reflected in so many books, plays, operas, and other musical pieces.[13] The sense of foreboding about TB also affected fashion; since the disease was associated with skinny, wan people, extra weight was regarded as healthful and attractive.

Tuberculosis has been present in human populations since the beginning of recorded history, and even before that, as indicated by the detection of tubercles on mummified remains in Asia and the Middle East. In the nineteenth century, however, it rose to become the number one cause of death. Statistically, it replaced smallpox, which was on the wane due to the introduction of vaccination, but TB might have surpassed all other diseases anyway, because it was so well suited to prosper in the Industrial Age. Though no one knew it at the time, TB was commonly spread through the coughing and spit of those affected. The close living conditions that resulted from the migration of workers to urban settings was a boon to TB. Even more than that, it benefited from the vast increase in travel brought by trains and steam navigation. Populations on the move, with people swirling past one another to all corners of the globe offer TB a statistically bountiful chance of finding new hosts. In fact, nothing helped the spread of TB more than the treatment normally prescribed for it: a vacation. Whether patients were seeking sea air, warm climates, or bracing mountain breezes, they hacked and coughed their way through mobbed stations and crowded compartments to get where they were going. Those sitting alongside TB victims thought nothing of it, and even the coughing was only considered an annoyance if it sprayed blood onto clean clothes. They just didn't know what was wrong.

On the evening of Friday, March 24, 1882, Robert Koch told them. He showed pictures of just exactly what tuberculosis is, in bacteria form. And on that first night of a new tide against TB, he told them how it spread and what could be done, as of that very moment, to stop it:

> Measures specifically directed against tuberculosis are not known to preventive medicine. But in future the fight against this terrible plague of mankind will deal no longer with an undetermined something, but with a tangible parasite, whose living conditions are for the most part known and can be investigated further. . . . First of all, the sources from which the infectious material flows must be closed as far as this is humanly possible. One of these sources, and certainly the most essential one, is the sputum of consumptives, whose disposal and change into a harmless condition has not thus far been accomplished. It cannot be connected with great difficulties to render such pthisical sputum harmless by suitable procedures of disinfection and to eliminate thereby the largest part of the infective tuberculous material.[14]

In frustration, Professor Cohn had once described the world of bacteria as "chaos." Koch's methods and his leadership brought order to the miasma. Embraced as a hero by the public, Koch offered hope that all contagious diseases could be trapped under the microscope, just as TB had. In very short order, they were. After a hundred centuries of hysteria, confusion, and superstition, the 1880s brought Koch's soft-spoken certainty to the understanding of contagious disease.

The very fact that germ theory did constitute a revolution disenfranchised some people, though Virchow remained ill-disposed toward it all of his life. So did Benjamin Ward Richardson, a famous English physician and an authority on anesthetics; he dismissed it as "research good enough in its way as a piece of natural history . . . but a positive insanity when accepted as the one absorbing pursuit . . . leading to Babel with its utter profusion of tongues and separating, for a time, our modern art of cure from the accumulated treasures of knowledge, wisdom, and light of over two thousand years."[15] Where TB was concerned, though, the light of two thousand years' learning was a small and flickering candle; it was Koch's bacteriology that lit the night.

Arthur Conan Doyle, who graduated from medical school in 1881, followed Koch's career avidly. Regarding the aftermath of the discovery of the tuberculosis bacterium, Doyle wrote, "Honours now crowded thick and fast upon the discoverer, but even as poverty had failed to drive him from his life's work, so the greater trial of success was unable to relax his diligence."[16]

In 1890, the German government sponsored a new research laboratory, the Institute for Infectious Diseases, tacitly built for its first director, Robert Koch. That same year, scientists gathered in Berlin for yet another momentous lecture by Koch; according to the rumors galloping through the city, he was going to make an epochal announcement.[17] In a grand hall called the Busch Circus, with seating for 8,000 and decorated to look like a Greek temple—a far cry from the reading room at the Physiological Society—Koch announced that as a natural outgrowth of his work with the TB bacteria, he had discovered a substance that slowed its growth, at least in early testing on animals. Whatever Koch said, the news flashed around the world that he had a cure for tuberculosis. From then on he was in the middle of a maelstrom, hailed a hero, besieged by desperate patients, decried by colleagues, and still trying to continue testing of the substance, which he called tuberculin. Koch was unsettled in his personal life at that juncture, since he was in the process of divorcing Emmy in favor of a young model, which may have contributed to his unfortunate decision to rush tuberculin testing in humans. The scientific controversy then became a very real human tragedy, as tuberculin was found to accelerate, rather than stop, the march of the disease. Tuberculin became known as "Koch's Poison," though it was later used successfully in testing for the presence of tuberculosis in humans.

For a few years in the early 1890s, Robert Koch was vilified for his role in producing tuberculin. Until his death in 1910, he remained heartbroken by the whole affair. He continued to pursue important work at the institute, some of it in concert with Paul Ehrlich, and in 1905, he received the second Nobel Prize awarded in Medicine and Physiology. Koch also traveled extensively, addressing public health problems in Africa and the Middle East.

The furor over tuberculin eventually faded, but even at its height, it couldn't remove Koch from his place in bacteriology. After March 24, 1882, that place was secure for all time.

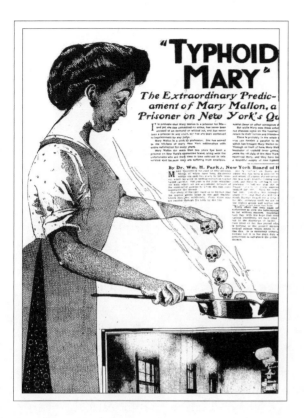

George A. Soper and
Mary Mallon
TRAILING DEATH

The motto of the New York City Department of Public Health in 1915 was rooted in realism—as was every person who survived more than a year or two on the job there. The department was charged with protecting the residents of New York City from the medical risks of life in a city crisscrossed by millions of people, billions of rodents and bugs, and trillions of germs. It wasn't as hard as it sounded, though. "Public health is purchasable," the department's motto declared. "Within natural limitations a community can determine its own death-rate."[1]

Normally, the cost was counted in dollars, and in 1915, the primary expenditures were for sanitation and education. However, that year, the public good exacted a slightly higher price. A woman named Mary Mallon, the first typhoid carrier to be directly linked to an epidemic, received a life sentence as a result of a medical anomaly and her own bad judgment. Miss Mallon saw herself only as a cook, earning an honest living. The New York Department of Public Health regarded her as the agent of a preventable epidemic and took steps to lock her away for good.

For centuries, people stricken with leprosy had been segregated from the general population under the threat of law. While leprosy is not easily communicable, it did cause an irrational fear. In our own time, Cuba established a policy early in the worldwide AIDS epidemic of segregating people with the disease or its precursor, the HIV infection.[2] The Cuban system, which did not leave patients with a choice, did provide them with pleasant surroundings and first-rate medical care. And it worked. In 1995, when the nearby islands of the Bahamas counted an infection rate of 131.4 cases per 100,000 and Bermuda counted 77.2, Cuba reported 0.8 cases.[3]

The policy in Cuba was controversial, despite its success in controlling the spread of the disease. "The price in terms of loss of human freedom is more than we are willing to pay," said a medical ethicist from the U.S., commenting on the Cuban system of incarceration.[4] Mary Mallon, infamous under the name she hated, "Typhoid Mary," paid that same price with the last twenty-three years of her life. Public health may well be purchasable, but it is the easy problems that require mere money.

In March of 1903, the city of Ithaca in the Finger Lakes region of New York State was in the midst of a typhoid epidemic that seemed utterly hopeless, with more than 1,200 people infected and dozens dying each week. "In point of fact, Ithaca is a very dirty town, full of ancient evils," wrote a resident named J. C. Bayles, who came to the conclusion that "on the basis of such a sanitary administration as Ithaca has become habituated to and has deemed sufficient, it might very well be four or five years before typhoid fever ceased to be epidemic in Ithaca."

In 1903, typhoid (or enteric) fever was one of the scourges of civilization, the eighth-greatest cause of death in the U.S. and third among diseases, behind tuberculosis and cancer.[5] Typhoid is liable to break out wherever people cluster, in country villages or big cities. In the nineteenth century, it periodically decimated the population of cities such as Philadelphia, Memphis, and New Orleans. With many different disguises, typhoid attacks people (animals are immune to it) along unpredictable lines. After incubating for one to three weeks, it usually starts to wreak havoc on a patient as a fever, followed by severe headaches, malaise, loss of appetite, and cramps. All of which might ebb and flow over several months. In some cases patients experience a spotted rash on the belly and nosebleeds, as well as even worse bleeding in the intestines. Not everyone dies as a typhoid outbreak runs its course; the average is about 7 to 14 percent of those infected (in the modern era, patients treated with antibiotics rarely die), but it doesn't necessarily prey on the weak, as some illnesses do. The Ithaca epidemic took the lives of twenty-seven Cornell University students between January and March 1903—one-and-a-half percent of the student body,[6] a higher proportion than the death rate for Ithaca as a whole.

Faced with "decimation if not extermination,"[7] the city hired Dr. George A. Soper, an independent consultant from New York City, and granted him dictatorial powers in combating the epidemic. Soper rushed to the scene. He was not a medical doctor but a civil engineer specializing in sanitation, chosen because typhoid fever is very often traced to contaminated water.

Soper was born in 1870 in New York City, where he eventually earned a doctorate in engineering from Columbia University. He was working for a filtration company in 1900 when the vicious hurricane known only as "The Storm" hit the city of Galveston, Texas. Soper was summoned to the scene and put in charge of implementing a sanitation system; his speedy work probably saved at least as many lives as the storm took in the first place.

A man of average build, Soper had a wide, high forehead and hooded eyes that seem foreboding even in old photographs. But then, nothing genteel or chipper could be expected of a man summoned to emergencies like a fireman—to confront not flames but the public at its dirtiest and most lazy. In Ithaca, Soper cleaned out contaminated creeks, removed standing water, and generally insisted that the residents clean up their city. Within a month, his measures succeeded in ending the typhoid epidemic, making him a celebrity in the state.

While Soper went on to become a specialist in stopping typhoid epidemics when they took hold in cities, minor outbreaks, affecting only small pockets of people, continued to be common occurrences. One such flare-up swept through the household of Charles Warren in 1906. Warren, a New York banker, was summering with his family in Oyster Bay, Long Island—a swank residential community that was enjoying newfound fame as the home of President Theodore Roosevelt.

Charles Warren leased a spacious, airy home in the town, hoping to spend a pleasant summer with his wife and daughters and a staff of servants. In June and July they had a fine time, but in late August, six of the eleven people in the household fell ill with typhoid fever: three family members and three servants. Even as they recovered, Charles Warren called in experts to look for the source of the fever. The water was tested and so was the milk supply, with no results. The fruit and vegetables in the household were likewise blameless.[8] The property did not have any standing water or a cesspool that might have harbored bacteria.

Once all six patients recovered fully, Charles Warren went away stymied, but the man who owned the house couldn't rest with the deadly mystery afoot. Aware that George Soper was regarded as the best typhoid detective in the country, he commissioned him to find the cause: a city-size investigator to work the problem in a single household. Hiring the great Dr. Soper was not a case of overreaction, not where typhoid fever was concerned. If the landlord worried that without a definite answer, the fever could flare up again without warning, he was right. But he couldn't have known just how right.

From Soper's point of view, the appeal of the Warren case was that it defied the reasoning of all previous assumptions about typhoid fever. The accepted doctrine was that people contracted typhoid from patients already suffering from the disease, or through media such as water, milk and food. Soper, however, believed that there was another alternative. "I had become interested in a theory concerning the transmission of typhoid other than that which was usually accepted," he explained.

Soper read the current literature on the subject of typhoid fever and was especially interested in a flurry of developments that took place in the wake of a speech by Robert Koch in November 1902.

Dr. Koch, Germany's eminent germ theorist, advanced his finding that typhoid could be communicated not only by current patients but also by convalescent ones. Almost simultaneously, Paul Frosch theorized that in some people exposed to typhoid, the infectious bacilli did not develop into an attack on the body but remained dormant in the intestines.[9] A person could have typhoid, technically, and never even know it. In a similar train of thought, a pair of German scientists named von Drigalski and Conradi proved in 1904 that people who had once been sick with typhoid but were entirely recovered from the symptoms might still be producing the bacilli many years later. Moreover, von Drigalski and Conradi identified several people who had been in contact with typhoid patients, developed no symptoms of their own, and yet produced the bacilli in their digestive tracts.[10]

Finally, another German physician, following the lead of von Drigalski and Conradi, examined 1,700 people who had never, to their knowledge, had typhoid fever. He found eleven who carried the bacilli.

Typhoid "carriers," as they came to be known, added a whole new element to the understanding of human illness. Apparently, people could play host to a disease without contracting it, a fact that vastly expanded the challenge of combating epidemics. The foe could be invisible—and was, in the case of typhoid carriers.

Even so, as of 1906, no example had been found of a healthy person actually having caused a typhoid outbreak. To the general public, the long tradition of medical knowledge still dictated that it was sick people, not well ones, who spread a disease. Only in the shrouded realm of the medical journals was the latest science saying otherwise. With those medical journals in mind, Soper set out to Oyster Bay in the winter of 1906. He intended to start right out testing the latest theory from Germany, but first he was tempted back to the old line of thinking. "I was led from the proper tack for a time by being informed that the family was extremely fond of soft clams and that supplies of these shell fish had frequently been obtained from an Indian woman who lived in a tent on the beach, not far from the house, and whose supplies of clams were sometimes taken from places that were not improbably polluted with sewage."[11] With raw sewage dumped into open waters, the ocean wasn't necessarily cleaner than any dirty creek that ran through a city slum. Because of that, typhoid fever was often traced to fresh seafood. In the case of the Warren family, though, Soper found that the last of the clams had been consumed too long before the typhoid outbreak to be the likely source. Anyway, the whole town was eating the woman's daily catch, and nobody outside of the Warren house became sick. The clams turned out to be a red herring. Soper reverted to his original intent and focused on the Warren residence.

"I started out by a careful investigation of the visitors' list for that Summer," Soper told a reporter, "I followed up the health record in so far as it included typhoid, of every person who had entered the house that season."[12] He was specifically looking for someone who had lived through typhoid fever at some earlier point, someone who might unknowingly still be carrying the bacillius and spreading the disease.

For a while, it seemed as though the Warrens had the healthiest circle of friends and acquaintances on Long Island. None of them had ever had typhoid fever, been exposed to it, or so much as looked at Ithaca on a map during the winter of '03. Soper continued to ask questions, though. While his investigation started a good three months after the outbreak, the Warren family tried valiantly to remember any arcane details that might have import. Finally, someone told Soper that the family had changed cooks on August 4—three weeks before the first case of typhoid in the household.

The time frame was just about right, although the family remembered the cook as a notably robust woman. She certainly hadn't been one of the ones to fall ill with typhoid. "The cook," Soper said, "was described as an Irish woman about forty years of age, intelligent, tall, heavy, single and noncommunicative. She seemed to be in perfect health. She was not known ever to have had an attack of typhoid."[13] However, the family did remember that on one particular occasion, she had prepared a treat of peaches and whipped cream for them. Normally, a cook would not have handled cold food, such as fresh fruit, but she was filling in that day for one of the serving girls. On hearing of the peaches Dr. Soper—being Dr. Soper—instantly pictured the cook handling them with poorly washed hands. Learning from the Warrens that her name was Mary Mallon, he insisted on seeing her.

To complicate matters, Mallon had quit the Warren household months before and her whereabouts were unknown. Even while Soper was trying to locate her, though, he traced her past work record through a number of employment agencies. No faithful old family retainer, Mallon had over the previous ten years held a long list of positions in houses throughout the Northeast. She was generally regarded as a fine chef, but brusque in personality.

As Soper wended his way through interviews with eight of the cook's former employers, he was stunned to learn that all but one of the households had suffered an outbreak of typhoid during, or soon after, her period of employment. The locales were far-flung—from Dark Harbor, Maine, to Tuxedo Park, New York—and in each case, the typhoid outbreak was isolated within the household. It was never part of a municipal occurrence. At one house, the one in Dark Harbor, only Mallon and the head of the household remained healthy during the typhoid outbreak; he was so grateful for her services in helping tend the others, he gave her a bonus of fifty dollars.

Interestingly enough, Soper found that the families themselves were not as helpful as they might have been. "Nearly all the epidemics which I was inquiring into," he said, "had been investigated soon after they occurred, and had been explained in a different way. The answers to my questions were therefore unconsciously framed so as to convince me that the original explanations were correct."[14]

Soper saw the bigger pattern, though, and urgently tried to

locate Mary Mallon before she could strike again, in her unwitting way. He was too late. When he finally found her, working in a residence on Park Avenue in New York, he also found a family deep in mourning. A daughter in the household had only just died of typhoid fever. A chambermaid was recovering from it. Dr. Soper lost no time in paying a visit to the family cook. "If she were implicated in the outbreaks it was, of course, innocently," he explained, "I supposed that she would be glad to know the truth and to be shown how to take such precautions as would protect those about her against infection. . . I hoped that we might work out together the complete history of the case and make suitable plans for the protection of her associates in the future."

Very little was ever known about Mallon's background, except that she was born in Ireland and was in her late thirties at the time Soper identified her. She didn't seem to have any relatives in America, though she did have a number of friends, including at least one beau, during the time that Soper sought her out.

Dr. Soper may not have been the most tactful person in the world, but he had been trained to believe that preparation could win the day. He believed in lining up his facts so tightly that there was no room for anything extraneous—such as opinion. Mary Mallon was his perfect opposite. With the survival instincts of the working class and the desperation of an immigrant, she looked straight past facts and arguments. The final result was her only reality, and her response to it was based on necessity, as she then saw it.

Dr. Soper recalled their meeting:

My interview was short. It started in the kitchen and ended almost immediately at the basement door. Reason, at least in the forms in which I was acquainted with it, proved unavailing. My point of view was not acceptable and the claims of science and humanity were unavailing. I never felt more hopeless.

The next interview was staged more deliberately. Mary

had a friend whom she often visited at night in the top of a Third Avenue tenement. He kindly offered to manage for the meeting and one night, after her work was done, I awaited her with a physician, Dr. Bert Hoobler . . . We waited at the head of the stairs in the Third Avenue house.

At length Mary Mallon came. Dr. Hoobler and I described the situation with as much tact and judgment as we possessed. We explained our suspicions. We pointed out the need of examinations which might reveal the source of the infectious matter which Mary was, to a practical certainty, producing. We wanted a small sample of urine, one of feces and one of blood.

Indignant and peremptory denials met our appeals. We were unable to make any headway. Mary's position was like that of the lawyer who, on being told by the judge that the facts were all against his client, said that he proposed to deny the facts. Mary denied that she was a carrier. She referred to the Dark Harbor outbreak for proof of her helpfulness and to the gift from her employer there as testimony of the same. Far from causing typhoid, she had helped to cure it. Nothing could alter her position. As Mary's attitude toward us at this point could in no sense be interpreted as cordial, we were glad to close the interview and get down to the street.[15]

If kicking and screaming and abject denial could stave off bad medical news, then Mary Mallon would never have been identified as a typhoid carrier. She would have gone on as a cook, a calling in which she was utterly happy, and would never have laid eyes on George A. Soper again. However, for all of Mary Mallon's pathetically childlike tantrums, she could not keep the New York City Department of Public Health from rounding her up in a paddy wagon (a test of strength that she lost against five policemen) and depositing her at a Detention Hospital, where she was tested against her will and found to be a prodigious source of typhoid bacilli. In fact, she produced as much as a patient in the acute stage of the disease.[16] Soper visited her at the Detention Hospital, but not to cheer her up or bring her flowers. On behalf of humanity, as he explained, he wanted to collect details about her medical history, so that doctors would have a better understanding of the typhoid-carrier phenomenon. In addition, he wanted to work with her in planning a course that might reverse her unique condition. To all of this, she didn't say a word. There was no more shouting. She just waited until he was finished talking and then locked herself in the bathroom.

Mallon did eventually tell someone at the hospital that she had never been sick with typhoid fever. She wouldn't discuss her background, though, or contact any family members. A few friends came to visit, but other than that, she was incarcerated just as though she had committed a crime. "The case of this woman brings up many interesting problems," said Dr. William H. Park, director of the bacteriological laboratory at the New York City Department of Health. Dr. Park wasn't referring to the many intriguing facts surrounding her epidemiology, though. "Has the city a right to deprive her of her liberty for perhaps her whole life?" he asked a meeting of the American Medical Association in 1908. "The alternative is to turn loose on the public a woman who is known to have infected at least twenty-eight persons."[17] And caused the death of one.

The newspapers didn't have much sympathy. They labeled her "Typhoid Mary" and her case became as well known in casual conversation as it was in medical societies. However, some people came to Mary Mallon's defense; a team of lawyers filed a suit on her behalf against the Department of Public Health, calling for her release. They weren't the only ones who believed that illness, however threatening to others, was no cause for the revocation of individual rights. To some people, germ theory itself was just another rationalization for government oppression.

"If one unfortunate woman must be labeled 'Typhoid Mary,' why not send her other companions?" suggested a writer from Newark in a letter to the editor dated June 30, 1909, more than two years after Mallon was first locked away. "Start a colony on some unpleasant island, call it 'Uncle Sam's Suspects,' there collect Measles Sammy, Tonsilitis Joseph, Scarlet Fever Sally, Mumps Matilda and Meningitis Matthew. Add Typhoid Mary, request the sterilized prayers of all religionized germ fanatics and then leave the United States to enjoy the glorious freedom of the American flag under a medical monarchy."[18]

During that summer in 1909, a New York Supreme Court Justice decided against Mallon's lawsuit.[19] By then, she had no companions, except a mongrel dog who was her only friend. Living in a cottage on the grounds of the North Brother Hospital, she was treated as though simply catching sight of her would cause instant death. A nurse brought meals three times a day and left them on the doorstep, hurrying away before Mallon could open the door. That, it seemed, was to be her fate for the rest of her life.

Oddly enough, some bacteriologists and other medical researchers took Mallon's side, on humanitarian grounds, even though they knew better than most people just what a serious threat she posed as a walking test tube of deadly germs. But she wasn't the only one. Research into the prevalence of typhoid carriers, in the aftermath of Mallon's incarceration, revealed that about one in thirty people who recovered from typhoid fever continued to host the bacillius and could potentially spread the disease. And then there were the other uninfected carriers, like Mary Mallon. One such case was found close on the heels of the Mallon investigation, when a man working in the Adirondacks as a guide was found to be the cause of an outbreak involving thirty-six people. "Typhoid John," as he was known, proved to be entirely cooperative, submitting not only to testing but to experimental treatment.[20] The most informed, humanitarian opinion in the Mallon case was that she was being unfairly singled out: There were an estimated 10,000 typhoid carriers in the United States alone. With changes in behavior, any of them could live in their own communities with no threat to others. So could Mary Mallon.

First, she would have to change her sloppy ways in the bathroom and wash her hands thoroughly and without fail. Second, she would have to use extreme care in many smaller details of hygiene, all of which had been explained to her. And third, she would have to stay out of kitchens forever. In terms of a profession, she could do practically anything she wanted—except handle food for other people. The rules were not that complicated, but nonetheless, no one in a position of authority wanted to be responsible for releasing her; it was easier to keep her on North Brother Island.

Then, in January 1910, the Department of Public Health welcomed a new commissioner, Dr. Ernst J. Lederle. The following month, he set Mary Mallon free.

"She has been released because she has been shut up long enough to learn the precautions that she ought to take," Dr. Lederle said in a statement. "I have taken a personal interest in her case and I am doing what I can for her. It seems to me that the people of this city ought to do something for her. She is a good cook and until her detention had always made a comfortable living. . . . I know where she is, but must decline to give any information on this point. She has promised to report to me regularly and not to take another position as a cook. I am going to do all I can to help her."[21]

The department initially arranged a job for Mallon as a laundress in New York, but having once reigned as a cook, she couldn't abide the lower status of the washtub. She quit, and within a few years her reports to the department trailed off.

Mallon might not have had her second chance at freedom elsewhere. In Germany and several other European countries, people found to be typhoid carriers were placed under strict police control, sometimes including incarceration.[22] Although the recognition of the carrier in the spread of typhoid fever was a major breakthrough in the first decade of the twentieth century, researchers of the day spent little time probing the reasons some people were prone to a long-term infection. Instead, typhoid research turned toward the creation of a vaccine. Since those who had had the disease were immune ever after (whether they continued to carry the bacilli or not), it seemed a conducive path. In 1914–15, the first typhoid vaccinations became available and showed promise, in time to save at least a few soldiers in World War I from a disease tailor-made to thrive in the filth of the trenches.

In January of 1915, an outbreak of typhoid fever swept through the Sloane Hospital for Women, a well-run maternity hospital in midtown Manhattan. The illness seemed to target the staff, though some of the patients were affected as well. During the weeks that followed, kitchen helpers took to teasing the cook, a Mrs. Brown, by calling her Typhoid Mary. By the time investigators from the Department of Public Health arrived on the scene to look for the source of the fever, Mrs. Brown was tired of the nickname, and she didn't like the implication of their visit. Overnight, she quit. Already suspicious, the investigators now focused all their efforts on finding her.

After several months, a policeman named John Bevins managed to trace Mrs. Brown to a home in the Queens borough of New York City. He watched from a distance as she entered the house. Though her face was covered by a veil, Bevins recognized her walk. He immediately called the Department of Health, notifying them that Mrs. Brown was unquestionably Mary Mallon. An automobile full of doctors and detectives rushed to the scene and ran up the steps of the house. Whoever was inside the house refused to answer their repeated knocks, calls, and poundings.

Someone found a ladder and the doctors climbed up to the second story, where they scrambled in through a window. Only then did Mrs. Brown–Mary Mallon give herself up.[23] Against her will, she was then returned to North Brother Island, still insisting that she didn't have typhoid or its germs and couldn't have been responsible for any epidemics.

"The story of Typhoid Mary indicates how difficult it is to teach infected people to guard against infecting others," observed Dr. Soper, after Mallon's second incarceration. "She knew that when she cooked she killed people and yet she deliberately sought employment as a cook in a hospital. Why did she do this?"[24]

As the record of the career of "Mrs. Brown" filled in, it was found that Mallon had created two other outbreaks before finding work at the hospital. In all, she caused fifty-seven known cases of typhoid, three of which ended in death.[25] It's hard to believe that at some point she didn't start to look past the coincidence of her association with typhoid. But her prowess as a cook was her pride, and to a great extent, her identity. Selfishly, she couldn't leave it behind. If there was another reason, or any other answer to the mystery of Mary Mallon, she never betrayed it. She spent the rest of her life on North Brother Island, strong-willed to the end, never confiding the story of her life to anyone. The only visitors she had were priests from St. Luke's Roman Catholic Church in Manhattan. At the time of her death in November 1938, a person familiar with her case wrote, "It is good to note that in later years she lost much of her bitterness and lived a fairly contented if necessarily restricted life."[26]

George Soper often lectured about his experience in recognizing Mary Mallon as a typhoid carrier, yet it wasn't even the most famous case with which he was associated. In 1912, after the *RMS Titanic* struck an iceberg and sank in the North Atlantic, Soper was drafted to make a study of ice floes in the region, in order to lower the chances of further collisions. He also served as one of the first directors of the American Cancer Society. He died in 1948.

Typhoid fever is still ravaging underdeveloped regions, with 16 million cases reported annually around the world, at a cost of 500,000 lives. After years of research, the vaccine is neither fully effective nor even practical in fighting a disease that can strike anywhere.

In 2002, however, medical researchers finally shed light on the reason that some people become typhoid carriers. The difference may lie not in the susceptibility of the human host but in the genetic structure of the bacteria to which they are exposed. According to research carried out jointly by scientists in England and Sweden, the typhoid bacillius normally contains an enzyme that interferes with the production of the so-called virulence factors, which promote a continuing presence within the organs of the body. The less common, long-term type of bacillius found in typhoid carriers has a mutant enzyme that does not do much in the way of interfering with the virulence factors. In a carrier such as Typhoid Mary, they can have their way and hold forth in the body indefinitely. "This is the first time that this type gene regulation has been linked with the carrier state of typhoid," said Dr. Jay Hinton, one of the researchers responsible for the finding. One small part of the Typhoid Mary mystery was solved—perhaps the only one that did not die with that most stubborn woman.

III
MAGIC BULLETS

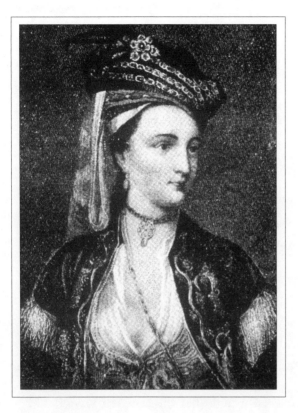

Lady Mary Wortley Montagu
WORLDLY WISE

When Lady Mary Montagu left London early in 1717 to live in Constantinople, the poet Alexander Pope was bereft, reflecting that he passed by her house "with the same Sort of Melancholy that we feel upon Seeing the Tomb of a Friend."[1] Pope was hopelessly in love with her at the time, but he wasn't the only one to respond to the excitement about Lady Montagu. She was a delicate, fine-featured young woman, an aristocrat and an heiress, but those were merely her inheritances. It was her highly original wit that made her celebrated. Underlying her sly humor was an erudition that brought her the respect of men and women alike, and made her a renowned conversationalist and correspondent.

When Lady Montagu wrote back to Pope, she was staying at a secluded resort near Constantinople favored by wealthy Christians in Islamic Turkey. Picking up on Pope's funereal theme, she wrote, "The Heats of Constantinople had driven me to this place, which perfectly answers the Description of the Elysian fields." After describing the glades and fountains that surrounded her villa there, she continued, "But what perswades me more fully of my Decease is the Situation of my own Mind, the profound Ignorance I am in of what passes amongst the Living, which only comes to me by chance, and the great Calmness with which I receive it."[2]

Lady Montagu was happier when she was out and about, on her own or with a guide, exploring Turkey's cities. Her husband was the

British ambassador to Turkey, but she looked upon their sojourn there as her opportunity just as much as his. Having learned Turkish, she often put on the veil and flowing garb worn by Islamic women, so that she could roam around and learn about the culture firsthand.[3] While she was in Adrianople, the capital of the Turkish Empire, she made it her business to watch a certain local custom purported to save people from contracting smallpox. Lady Montagu's curiosity about that custom—inoculation—and her influence in promoting it would help to save millions of people in Europe and the Americas from death due to smallpox in the eighteenth century. While she was not the only person to figure in the introduction of inoculation into Western medicine, she was its crucial proponent, the first European to accept fully the topsy-turvy idea that in order to avoid smallpox, one has to seek out and contract smallpox.

Lady Mary Pierrepont was born in 1689, the daughter of the Earl of Kingston and the granddaughter, through her mother's side, of the Earl of Denbigh. Her mother died when she was only four, after giving birth to a baby boy. Lady Mary was an unusually studious girl, taking it upon herself to read widely and even to learn Latin. Several of her father's prominent friends, including the playwright William Congreve, encouraged her studies, taking time to converse with her in Latin. Her relationship with her father, however, was not always as cordial. The headstrong girl and her dour father had a tendency to infuriate each other. For a time, Lady Mary professed an intention to remain unmarried and devote herself to study, a plan the Earl accepted, perhaps because it meant that his fortune would stay in his own family. After she began to show an interest in a beau, Edward Wortley Montagu—who was very rich but wouldn't sign an acceptable prenuptial agreement—her father arranged a marriage with an Irishman who was more acceptable in every way, to him, at least. As to Mary, she eloped with Wortley.

Lady Montagu, as she was known after the marriage, was unquestionably a beautiful teenager, with a creamy complexion along with the oval face and petite features that seemed to signal good breeding in the eighteenth century. For three years, she was an insouciant young bride, working on her writings and making herself popular in London society. Because of the elopement, Lady Montagu was estranged from her father, but that didn't concern her much. The only true tragedy of that period of her life was the death of her younger brother at the age of twenty, from smallpox. Then, in December 1715, she contracted the same disease. She wrote in a verse describing herself at the time, "Beauty is fled, and spirit is no more." As she sank, her chances of recovery seemed grim.

"Smallpox was always present," the eighteenth-century historian Thomas Macauley wrote in *The History of England from the Accession of James II* [1685], "filling the churchyard with corpses,tormenting with constant fear all whom it had not yet stricken."[4] The disease, for which there was (and is) no cure[5] is an infection caused by a virus called variola. It emerged with the first human settlements in about 10,000 B.C. and was spread, person to person, for millennia afterward. Animals and insects can't be blamed; it was passed through the breath, the bodily fluids, or the clothes and bedding of humans.

About one third of those who contracted smallpox died from it, though the death rate was twice that in some outbreaks. The wonder is that civilization survived it at all. An epidemic in A.D. 180 killed approximately 5 million people in the Roman Empire, a disaster from which it never recovered. The scourge was liable to strike anywhere that two people met, but it descended on cities in epidemics that were especially hard on infants. During the eighteenth century, Berlin recorded a 2 percent survival rate among children under the age of five who contracted smallpox.

Because cleanliness and general health have no effect on the incidence of smallpox, its history can be traced in terms of the monarchs who were killed by it. Emperor Marcus Aurelius was one of those who died in the Roman epidemic in A.D. 180. But it struck all over the world, claiming Ciutláhuac, emperor of the Aztec empire (1520); the King and Queen of Ceylon and all of their sons

(1582); Emperor Ferdinand IV of Austria (1654); Emperor Fu-Lin of China (1661); Louis I of Spain (1724); and Czar Peter II of Russia (1730), among many others.[6] The deaths of those less famous were counted only in statistics.

Smallpox typically ran a course of about a month, starting with a two-week incubation period during which there were no symptoms. The illness then appeared in the form of a high fever, nausea, and aches, especially in the limbs. Within a few days, a rash would break out in and around the mouth, spreading to the rest of the body and then giving rise to bumps. At that time, the fever often returned, causing death. If the patient survived, the bumps turned into pustules: cones of flesh and fluid that felt hard inside, as though they contained a pea. Within a few weeks, the pustules scabbed over and fell off. Once the scabs were gone, the illness was over too, and at that point, patients would take stock. If they could see, they braced themselves for a look in the mirror. The only consolation was that they almost certainly wouldn't contract smallpox ever again. However, many who recovered were left blinded, and nearly everyone's skin was marked with pitting and redness. Often, the pitting was so extensive that the facial structure could be affected, causing crooked hollows in the cheeks and sagging scars on the chin or forehead. Those were the prospects that Lady Mary Montagu contemplated as she lay in her sickbed.

Lady Montagu's illness gave London's wags something to talk about for weeks. News of her surprising recovery obviously pleased her friends, but her more wicked acquaintances speculated on the effect that the pocks would have on her famed face, pausing over the news that her pustules had been *very* full. And deep.

Alexander Pope commemorated Lady Montagu's reappearance in London society by mentioning her in a poem, "Epistle to Jervas," referring to her as "a beauty whose eyes other beauties shall envy." They might well envy her eyes. But though she still presented an ideal from a distance, on closer view her face gave her away. In appearance, she was no longer one of London's goddesses, but only another of its smallpox victims. Her complexion was pitted and pocked. As Robert Halsband, her biographer, commented, "Her reputation henceforth was mainly that of a wit."[7]

Only the year before, an article about a peculiar smallpox preventative had appeared in the Royal Society of London's publication, *Philosophical Proceedings,* a general scientific journal that included medical news. The author was Dr. Emanuel Timoni, an Italian who had earned his medical degree at the University of Padua. Before moving permanently to Constantinople, he had lived in England, studying at Oxford University and even becoming a member of the Royal Society. In 1714, he wrote a letter to his fellow members that was eventually published under the title "An Account, or History, of the Procuring of the Small Pox by Incision, or Inoculation; As it has for Some Time Been Practised in Constantinople."[8] The Royal Society took his description seriously enough to commission another member to investigate it further. The second report was published in 1716, and inspired new discussions about smallpox, but little else for the time being.

Lady Montagu probably did not read the letters about smallpox in the *Philosophical Proceedings,* though she did meet Timoni in Constantinople, since he was the physician for the ambassador's family. Whether or not she spoke to him about her interest in smallpox is not certain, though it seems likely. They were both thinking about it quite actively during the same time span in the mid-1710s. And as soon as they met, it would have been sadly obvious to him that she had been stricken by the disease.

Whether Lady Montagu was inspired by Timoni or by her own new knowledge of Turkish culture, she made arrangements to investigate for herself the Turkish method of eradicating smallpox. In 1717, she wrote to one of her friends in England about what she'd seen. "A propos of Distempers," she began, "I am going to tell you a thing that I am sure will make you wish your selfe here. The Small Pox so fatal and so general amongst us [in England] is here entirely harmless."

No statement could have been more astonishing to someone in Europe, where smallpox was anything but harmless. Lady Montagu continued:

There is a set of old Women who make it their business to perform the Operation. Every Autumn in the month of September, when the great Heat is abated, people send to one another to know if any of their family has a mind to have the small pox. They make partys for this purpose and when they are met (commonly 15 or 16 together) the old Woman comes with a nutshell full of the matter of the best sort of small-pox and asks what veins you please to have open'd. She immediately rips open that you offer to her with a large needle (which gives you no more pain than a common scratch) and puts into the vein as much venom as can lye upon the head of her needle, and after binds up the little wound with a hollow bit of shell, and in this manner opens 4 or 5 veins.[9]

The recipients of the pox, typically children, would go and play. After a few days, they might suffer a slight fever and a few spots, but once they were over that, they could consider themselves immune. "You may believe I am very well satisfy'd of the safety of the Experiment since I intend to try it on my dear little Son," Lady Montagu wrote to her friend. A person of fiercesome opinions, she then continued, "I am Patriot enough to take pains to bring this usefull invention into fashion in England, and I should not fail to write to some of our Doctors very particularly about it if I knew any one of 'em that I thought had Virtue enough to destroy such a considerable branch of their Revenue for the good of Mankind . . . Perhaps if I live to return I may, however, have courrage to war with 'em."[10]

Within the retinue that traveled with the Montagu family to Turkey was a surgeon (at that time, a surgeon held a lower rank than a physician) named Charles Maitland. In March 1718, Lady

Montagu directed Maitland to "engraft" smallpox into her son, Edward Junior, according to the Turkish method. Maitland blanched at the prospect of giving a deadly disease to his little charge, but he had no choice, as he later related:

> The Ambassador's ingenious Lady, who had been at some Pains to satisfy her Curiosity in this Matter, and had made some useful Observations on the Practice, was so thoroughly convinced of the Safety of it, that *She* resolve'd to submit *her* only Son to it, a very hopeful boy of about Six Years of Age.[11]

An elderly Greek woman was brought in to consult. And at Maitland's insistence, two physicians, probably including Timoni, were on hand to observe—in case the boy died. The only person who wasn't the least bit worried was Lady Montagu. As to her husband, he was away. About a week later, she wrote to him to explain what happened. "The boy was engrafted last Tuesday," she reported, "and is at this time singing and playing and very impatient for his supper."[12]

In making the decision to inoculate Edward Jr., Lady Montagu took a step that very few Europeans had ever taken. The responsibility was hers, not only for using her son in an initial trial of inoculation but for breaking with her own culture to do so. She was a pioneer—willing in her heart to risk everything, but guided entirely by her intellect. Acting on the basis of both at once required a cool courage that indicates why she was just the person to lead a campaign on the wisdom of inoculation.

After returning to London with her husband and family, Lady Montagu waged her promised war on smallpox, even while sidestepping the medical profession that she suspected would get in the way. She worked a faultless plan, first generating publicity, then gaining the support of influential people, and finally engaging an unparalleled endorser: Caroline, the Princess of Wales and future Queen of England. The launch, so to speak, was in April 1721, when Lady Montagu summoned Mr. Maitland to London from his new post in the country and asked him to inoculate her four-year-old daughter. At least a half-dozen doctors were invited to watch, one of them being Sir Hans Sloane, who was no less than the King's physician.[13] The procedure went just as expected, both at the time and in the weeks following.

Londoners started out by talking about the bizarre chance that Lady Montagu had taken, but with encouraging words from the physicians who had seen the inoculation, the outrage faded and word was soon spreading that a way had actually been found to defend against the scourge of smallpox. Lady Montagu pressed forward, contributing anonymous articles about the innovation to the newspapers, and discussing it within her circle. One of those she seemed to convince was Princess Caroline, whose family had been through more than its share of smallpox funerals. In a sense, royal families had even more to lose than ordinary families from the disease. Where other parents lost a child, which was sorrow enough, royals lost an heir and, in some cases (like that of the Stuarts), a dynasty. Princess Caroline became intrigued with the idea of inoculation, but she wasn't quite ready to submit her own two daughters to any needles.

To arrange a test, the royal family offered pardons to six prisoners headed for the gallows if they would agree to be inoculated, or "variolated," as the process became known. Three men and three women were selected. All swore that they had never had smallpox before, since that would make them naturally immune. Apparently, one lied about that,[14] but he was, after all, sitting on death row. In any case, all six prisoners survived. Furthermore, one of the women agreed to continue the test, traveling at court expense to a town in the midst of a smallpox epidemic. She helped to care for victims, even sleeping in the same bed with an affected child, without becoming sick herself.

After more trials, including one involving the students at a charity school, Caroline agreed to have her two daughters variolated. With that, the idea spread quickly. As is the case with almost any medical breakthrough, though, many people found reasons to oppose the idea. The role of Lady Mary Montagu and Princess Caroline in promoting inoculation angered chauvinists, one minister dismissing them in print as "a few Ignorant Women, amongst an illiterate and unthinking People."[15] But critics received their best ammunition from reports of deaths due to variolation. The process was never perfectly safe, as Lady Montagu had thought when she first saw it used in Turkey. At best, it was a percentage play. The odds of dying from variolation were not nearly as great as those of dying from smallpox.

For a year or two, Lady Montagu continued to push for universal acceptance of smallpox inoculation and blamed the medical profession for slowing its progress, writing that physicians had "deluded" patients into fearing it so that they could continue to collect fees for treating the disease. The same charge would hound the profession for almost a hundred years.

After leaving the fight against smallpox to others, Lady Montagu continued to be a well-known personality, though an unsettled one. By turns, she separated from her husband, reconciled with her father, and watched as Alexander Pope's love for her turned vitriolic. She also grew to reject her beloved but scandal-ridden son, Edward Junior. All were part of a slippery parade of people and emotions that led her to become cheerfully detached from close relationships by the time of her death, from cancer, in 1761.

When Edward Jenner discovered at the end of the century that cowpox—a very mild disease similar to smallpox—could be used effectively to inoculate against the more serious disease, he faced just as much opposition as had "the few Ignorant Women" who preceded him in the battle against smallpox. Eventually, "vaccination," as his form of inoculation was called (from the Latin for "cow"), was accepted, of course, and Jenner was hailed a hero. Because the risk from vaccination was much lower than that from variolation, it proved more popular in the long run. Even so, the war on smallpox would last another 180 years. But mankind finally won. On May 8,

1980, the World Health Assembly officially declared that the human race was free of smallpox. It was a momentous achievement for medical science. Variolation and vaccination had simply eradicated the virus from the planet—except for one thing.

Living cultures of the variola virus were retained by U.S. government at the Centers for Disease Control and Prevention in Atlanta and by the Russian Institute for Viral Preparations in Moscow. If either sample was accidentally released, an epidemic was sure to follow. Because vaccinations had been suspended by most countries in the 1970s, modern populations had little or no immunity. Inexplicably, the two governments repeatedly refused calls from international groups to destroy the virus, once and for all. A lot of people like to save things, just in case, but there was no reason not to destroy the stocks of humanity's worst enemy, the variola virus. After the terrorist attacks by Islamic extremists in 2001 and a subsequent series of deadly incidents with anthrax in the mail system, the U.S. government suggested that a terrorist group might have found a way to steal some of the smallpox virus from one of the two known repositories. If so, then it could be used as a very deadly weapon. Vaccinations for smallpox were renewed on a limited basis.

The truly glorious accomplishment is that smallpox was successfully eradicated as a disease, in an effort helped along by the agitation of Lady Mary Montagu. Whether it has, in fact, been reborn as a form of murder is a question for another chapter of human history.

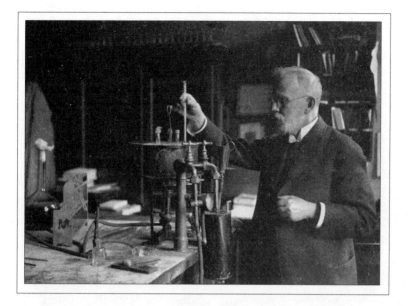

Paul Ehrlich
TAG OOK

I n all of the many articles published by *The New York Times* in late 1910 heralding Dr. Paul Ehrlich's stunning new medical cure, not one mention was made of just what exactly had been cured. The clearest reference was to "a malady which has been the scourge of the human race for centuries."[1] That narrowed the list of possibilities by approximately one disease: Radiation poisoning hadn't been around for centuries. But as of 1910, practically every other malady had been. Readers had to learn the name of the disease in the street, which was also, coincidentally, where they could contract it.

Even the word "syphilis" made people wince in the 1800s and early 1900s. Those who used slang ducked the real name and called it "the pox." Great newspapers weren't even that specific. The only ones who were long past squeamishness about syphilis were doctors who were inundated with patients—and staffers at insane asylums, which were bulging with syphilitic cases. A 1915 study in the United States reported that:

Syphilis infects about 5 to 10 percent of the adult population
Syphilis causes about 20 percent of all insanity
Syphilis causes many of the idiotic and feeble-minded children[2]

Other early twentieth-century studies contended that one third of insane asylum inmates were victims of syphilis.[3] A 1911 War

Department report acknowledged that 25 percent of the men in the Navy had venereal disease; while gonorrhea was the most prevalent, syphilis was a strong second. The Army was only a little better. Some regiments, though, had infection rates as high as 50 percent. While the U.S. Armed Forces were regarded as the worst in the world in the incidence of venereal disease,[4] across total populations, America was only average. Many European nations had an infection rate above 10 percent among adults.

Moralists liked to imply that syphilis, which is usually transmitted sexually, was a disease of the lower classes. But it is much more likely that it spread itself proportionally among the rich and the poor. The only difference is that since syphilis had many different symptoms, people with respectability to protect could label syphilis with any number of different names.

The most famous victim of the disease was Britain's Lord Randolph Churchill, the father of Sir Winston Churchill. In the midst of a sky-rocketing political career, his behavior turned erratic and even violent. Finally, he was committed to an asylum; the cause was late-stage syphilis. Many families, royal, noble, or peasant, had a similar secret.

In 1910, Dr. Paul Ehrlich of Frankfurt, Germany, gave them all hope, introducing a compound designed to eradicate syphilis but not the person carrying it. All previous cures had tended to do either both or neither. Dr. Ehrlich's expression for a chemical tailored to destroy a very specific microbe within the body, which is after all teeming with them, was a "magic bullet." Fired into a field crowded with targets, it would find just the right bull's-eye. When Dr. Ehrlich took aim at syphilis, the bullet he found was called Salvarsan. He also found that a great many people didn't want the world to have a cure for syphilis.

Like other sexually transmitted diseases, syphilis is carried in body fluids. The culprit is a form of bacteria, *Treponema pallidum,* that erupts within a few weeks of the initial exposure into a sore. After a couple of weeks, the initial sore goes away, giving rise to the light-hearted hope that it was nothing after all. Then the syphilis makes its appearance as a rash on the palms and feet, and sometimes all over the body. Other mild symptoms, such as a mild fever or fatigue, may come along, too; in fact, all of the symptoms may come and go, but they're completely gone after about two years. Once they disappear, patients are no longer contagious and some never show any further signs of syphilis.

Some people, however, after a break that can last up to forty years, display a new stage of many different and more serious symptoms, which is why syphilis was known as "the great imitator."[5] The most thorough diagnostician can be fooled by its ability to affect almost any organ. Even today, doctors often cannot easily diagnose syphilis; the great imitator has too many tricks. It can attack the nervous system, the heart, the bones, the eyes, or other parts of the body. A hundred years ago, doctors could only treat the symptoms, usually with frustrating results if *T. pallidum* was the root of the problem.

Syphilis seems to have been unknown in Europe before the late 1400s. It spread so rapidly at that point that no one was really certain where it came from, though there were many who were willing to cast aspersions. It was known variously as the Venetian disease, the Naples disease, and the French disease,[6] but not of course in Venice, Naples, and France, respectively. While the Europeans were playing pushball with the blame, the key to the origin of syphilis may have been the date at which it appeared. The last decade of the fifteenth century was the time of Columbus's first trip to the New World. Two archeologists, Bruce and Christine Rothschild, have recently found skeletal evidence that the disease was present in pre-Columbian cultures. Apparently, America was not the only thing that Columbus and his men discovered in 1492. However syphilis entered Europe, it ravaged cities, armies, and whole populations.

Syphilis was poorly understood during most of its first four hundred years in the Old World. All that was really known was that it spread primarily through sexual contact. For that reason, doctors made the erroneous assumption that it was closely related to gonorrhea; in putting that idea to rest through a series of experiments, a

French scientist took the first important step in syphilitic research in 1837. The treatment typically prescribed in the 1800s was the absorption of mercury through the sores. Mercury is a poison, of course, and doctors tried hard not to give their patients enough to hurt them, only enough to cure the disease. In any case, it rarely did much more than bring on the symptoms of mercury poisoning.

The spread of syphilis was probably responsible for those "Victorian morals," which seem so constricting to people who look back on them from a distance. During the nineteenth century, as syphilis proliferated at all levels of society, it changed in the public perception from a "carnal scourge," which might be shrugged off as another element in the world of illicit sex, to a "family poison"[7] destroying the innocent. That was something that no decent person could ignore. In a typical scenario, a man (the onus was unquestionably on the males) would contract syphilis before marriage but refrain from telling his new bride, either through ignorance of his own condition or carelessness about the risk. Not only would the wife almost certainly contract the disease, but so might any infants she bore. Because syphilis was so prevalent, the risk of contracting it with even one act of folly was very real. Those Victorian morals that tried to protect individuals and families from the disease sprang less from high-handed hypocrisy, as has often been the charge, and more from practicality.

Because syphilis still carries a social stigma, people generally avoid the topic and forget what a brutal social force it once was. A few historians have detected the beginnings of the feminist movement in the campaign that rose up against syphilis—and those beastly men who brought it home. Of course, wives could be beasts, too, in that sense. At the time, though, it was a segment of the female population that was motivated to protest.

While syphilis loomed over turn-of-the-century society as a social disease, its physiological properties remained a scientific mystery—one that began to crack open, a bit, with identification in 1905 of the microbe responsible for the disease. One of the reasons it took so long to recognize the cruel little bug was that it resisted stains—the dyes that microbiologists use to distinguish the various inhabitants of the microscopic world. Without stain, the syphilis bug had little definition and blended in with the background on a slide. Finally two German scientists, Fritz Schaudinn and Erich Hoffmann, captured it in their sights. At first, the elusive squiggle was called *Spirochaeta pallida,* a name that described its spiral shape. Later, when it was categorized as a treponemal microbe, its name was changed to *Treponema pallidum.* In 1906, another German scientist, August von Wassermann, followed up by cornering the microbe, announcing a test to discern its presence.

These two developments fit perfectly with Dr. Paul Ehrlich's plans, and almost certainly accelerated them. In 1906, he moved into a brand-new research institution, launched to accommodate his myriad interests in the field of medical research. Naturally, Dr. Ehrlich would be the director, and his first priority, so he announced, was the study of venereal diseases in hopes of finding cures.[8]

Paul Ehrlich was born in 1854 in a small town near Breslau (now called Wroclaw) in the region of Silesia in what is now southwestern Poland. Then it was part of Germany, or to be exact, East Prussia. Breslau has obviously seen its share of history, not to say maps, since 1854. Geography aside, Ehrlich regarded himself as a German throughout his life. Breslau offered a number of diversions worthy of a much larger European city, including a botanical park and an extensive zoo that opened in 1865, just in time to delight an eleven-year-old like Paul Ehrlich.

Paul's father, a rather odd man, was an innkeeper, or at least he held that title, while Mrs. Ehrlich kept the inn. Having high aspirations for her family, she insisted that her son Paul have a first-rate education that included college. A cousin in the family was a distinguished researcher, yet college still would have been an unusual goal for a middle-class family in the early 1870s, especially in view of the fact that Paul was no genius, at least not in the eyes of his teachers, who handed him grades that were barely average. Mrs.

Ehrlich must have known something, though. Where others saw a kid who couldn't memorize very well, she somehow saw the man who wouldn't have to. After high school, Ehrlich attended the University of Breslau, founded in 1702. It was composed of four undergraduate schools, representing various professions; Paul Ehrlich enrolled in the medical school.

Ehrlich was still not much of a student, yet he was committed to his own private research projects. He was especially interested in extending the use of stains in microscope slides, a complicated pursuit, but one made easier by the proximity of Germany's steadily advancing chemical industry. The art of staining involved finding dyes that would attach themselves only to certain microbes and then color them; later, Ehrlich and others who laid the groundwork for the development of antibiotics looked for chemicals that would attach themselves only to certain microbes—and kill them. Once, while Ehrlich was in a laboratory at the school working away, one of those other pioneers came through on a visit, accompanied by a professor. The visitor was Dr. Robert Koch, then an obscure research-physician from Wollstein, not far from Breslau. He was at the university to demonstrate his research on anthrax. When Koch paused in the lab to watch what Ehrlich was doing, the professor offered an introduction of sorts: "That is 'Little Ehrlich,'" he said, "He is very good at staining, but he will never pass his examinations."[9]

He was right—but only in his description of Ehrlich, who was little, even slight in build. Throughout his life, he regarded meals as an annoying interruption and often skipped them. However, he was not without his indulgences, and was rarely seen without a cigar. Ehrlich had sharp features and wore a well-trimmed beard that became the most noticeable characteristic of his face. His personality was less easily inventoried than his rather plain appearance. Paul Ehrlich was easygoing and almost always friendly when approached, even at work. His sense of humor hovered over most of his conversations, in the form of little jokes thrown out as asides. He had a particular habit of relaxing tense situations by making self-deprecating remarks.

People didn't always understand Ehrlich's odd jokes, but it was hard not to respond to the spirit behind them.

Ehrlich communicated in his own language of humor, but he also had his own language—literally. Martha Marquardt worked with Ehrlich for fifteen years and wrote a book about him after his death. She pointed out that he may have inherited the habit of creating new words from his father, who sometimes spent whole afternoons sitting by a window making up sentences out of his own words. Marquardt compiled a short glossary of Paul Ehrlich-speak, with some words based on actual German and some of his own creation. Of the latter, Marquardt gave several examples, including "Tag ook":

> His friendly "Tag ook" in which the "g," according to the Silesian idiom, was pronounced very hard, had quite another meaning than one would think it had. It was not merely "good morning" or "good day," but it was like a welcoming greeting saying "how nice that you have come," pleased to see you," and he had this kind "Tag ook" for everybody who came in to see him.[10]

According to Marquardt's recollections of conversations over the years, Ehrlich also tossed it into the middle of sentences for sake of sounding a friendly note or simply to fill in the rhythm of a long line of words. Perhaps it was a mantra of self-assurance, part of Ehrlich's puckish way of getting along in the world outside of his own thoughts.

By the time Ehrlich neared graduation, the opinion of him had changed and few people doubted that he had the ability to succeed. His senior thesis was, of course, on the subject of staining. It offered so much valuable new research that it was being widely discussed in Germany even before he left the university. However, there is always more to success than mere ability, and that was especially true of the scientific-medical community of Germany in the late nineteenth- and early twentieth centuries. There were two routes to success and the freedom to chart one's own course of research. The first lay with a professorship at a university; the second was a position at one of Germany's government-sponsored research institutions. Life in either one could be a test of survival, filled with sneak attacks and slow-acting poison. The fact that both the stakes and pressures were unnaturally high was reflected in the high rate of suicide among accomplished scientists. Even the smallest things mattered: In Germany during that era, conduct was carefully proscribed according to an unwritten system called *Standesgemäss,* which dictated how a person in each class and position should behave in social situations.[11]

Ehrlich was invariably polite, but he couldn't adopt the formality of *Standesgemäss* or indulge in the social climbing it encouraged. In that, his character may have been admirable, but it wouldn't help him in the world of German science.

Upon graduating with his medical degree in 1878, Ehrlich was immediately offered a post at the Charité Hospital in Berlin, working under Friedrich Theodor Frerichs, who was not only medical director of the hospital but personal physician to Otto von Bismarck, Germany's chancellor. For eight years, Ehrlich didn't even know how lucky he was to be reporting to a supportive man like Frerichs. Given unusual latitude by his new mentor, Ehrlich focused much of his time on a study of the white corpuscles of the blood; his observation of three distinct types has served as the basis of blood analysis ever since. He also worked on ways to test blood for the presence of typhoid fever.

While Ehrlich was at Charité, he married a woman named Hedwig Pinkus. They were very happy together and it was to be a successful marriage. It may be invidious to add that Hedwig also had a very large fortune.

In 1885, Dr. Frerichs had finally had enough of the pressures he had battled so long at the Charité. He killed himself by drinking a flask of an opium compound.[12] Frerichs's replacement immediately canceled Paul Ehrlich's projects and put him to work doing menial tasks. Ehrlich felt he had no choice but to quit, even though he had no real place to go.

Ehrlich was well qualified either to be a professor or to work in a government research institution, but he couldn't hope for either type of job. He was Jewish, and appointments of power were denied to Jews in Germany. Ehrlich didn't practice his religion actively, but even so, he wouldn't forsake it. He declined to undergo, even in a perfunctory way, the rite of baptism that would have cleared the way for him professionally.

After resigning from the Charité, Ehrlich set up his own research laboratory in a house on the outskirts of Berlin. Hedwig underwrote the expenses. Robert Koch, for one, thought it absurd that a researcher of such high stature had to work out of a homemade lab. Koch, now reigning as the director of the Institute for Infectious Diseases, had come a long way since he'd first met Ehrlich in Breslau. Yet because of the official constraints, the best that he could offer Ehrlich was an unpaid position. For the chance to work with Koch, Ehrlich became a docent, at least in name, and the two became close friends even as they notched a series of important achievements, together and separately. Among many other activities, Ehrlich made substantive improvements to an antitoxin for diphtheria that had been originated by another scientist at the institute, Emil von Behring. They duly formed a partnership to divide the profits from the cure, but Ehrlich came to feel cheated by Behring, both in money and professional respect. At the end of the 1890s, he was once again looking for a home for his research. Like Arrowsmith in the Sinclair Lewis novel of that name, he was forced to roam, looking for a place to save humanity without being entangled in it.

Friedrich Althoff, a government official in the industrial city of Frankfurt, stepped up to become Ehrlich's champion. In part because the chemical industry recognized that Ehrlich could lead it into the burgeoning field of pharmaceuticals,[13] the city of Frankfurt pressed hard for the creation of a new entity, the Institute for Experimental Therapy. Sponsored by the government, it opened in 1899 with Ehrlich as director. Perhaps because the institute had only just been built, or because Herr Althoff was a powerful ally, Ehrlich's religion did not hold him back. As busy as he was there, though, he longed to devote more time to chemotherapy, a term he coined for the sophisticated drugs he wanted to aim at the body's various maladies. As a matter of fact, Ehrlich was ahead of his time in believing that there were chemical cures for all of the diseases that attack the body, if researchers could only find them, understand them, and tag them. To that end, Althoff intervened again, encouraging a wealthy family in Frankfurt to sponsor a private research institute for Ehrlich. The result was the Georg Speyer Haus for Chemotherapy.

Between the two institutes, Ehrlich had an embarrassment of laboratories as outlets for his roving curiosity. In his mind, though, the division was clear. The Institute for Experimental Therapy concentrated on serumology, in which, as Ehrlich wrote, "the protecting substances of the body are products of the organism itself." Though that was preferable, according to Ehrlich, it was not always feasible. "In these cases," he explained, "chemotherapy must be used."[14] That was the focus at Speyer Haus.

Dr. Ehrlich set an early priority at Speyer Haus on finding a cure for syphilis. He selected it, in part, because *Spirochaeta pallida* was fairly large for a microbe, and very unique. Many other infectious diseases were caused by bacteria that were not only small and hard to detect but also vexingly similar to harmless microbes. Syphilis offered a big target for a magic bullet. In addition, it was a major scourge, which made a possible cure far more than just an engaging scientific problem. It was a chance to make a real difference in millions of lives. More pragmatically, syphilis was a dominant disease, and finding a way to eradicate it would make a real difference in the life of a fledgling institute.

Dr. Ehrlich led a team methodically through an investigation of more than six hundred compounds he thought might have promise, based on his previous experience. Concentrating especially on chemicals related to arsenic, Ehrlich oversaw extensive tests on 606 substances from 1905 to 1907. He had high hopes for the last one, but one of his assistants reported that it had not been effective. According to the assistant, No. 418 was the most promising of the lot. Ehrlich wasn't convinced; he didn't think that the test mechanism they were using was capable of delivering clear results. The syphilis program was temporarily suspended.

Ehrlich turned his attention to other things, such as collecting a Nobel Prize for Medicine in 1908, in honor of his contributions to immunology. It turned out to be that rare case when the prize was awarded to a person whose best work still lay ahead.

At Speyer Haus, many of the researchers came from outside of Germany; the list included many Americans over the years. Several Japanese scientists also worked there, most of them on leave from the Kitasato Institute for Infectious Diseases in Tokyo. Dr. Sahachiro Hata was on the staff at that institution in 1905, when he read of the isolation of *Spirochaeta pallida* by Schaudinn and Hoffmann. Hata immediately changed the direction of his own research, devising a method of cultivating *S. pallida* microbes in rabbits through inoculation. That was a skill Ehrlich admired, and in 1909, Hata arrived in Frankfurt by previous arrangement and presented himself to Dr. Ehrlich.

At their first meeting, Hata and Ehrlich had a protracted politeness contest, with the exchange of many bows and *tag ooks*. When they were both finally tapped out, Ehrlich turned to business and handed Hata two little bottles, containing compounds "418" and "606." With that he asked him to test all of the substances previously collected, using syphilitic rabbits as subjects. "So happy, Herr Professor," Dr. Hata replied. That was before he saw the 604 other little bottles.

However, Dr. Hata was as thorough a researcher as Ehrlich himself. His final report that No. 606 was "very efficacious" charged Speyer Haus with excitement. Further testing, including a program involving human patients, confirmed the first results.

On April 19, 1910, Dr. Ehrlich addressed the Congress for Internal Medicine, which convened in Germany that year. His speech was warmly anticipated and many physicians came to the assembly hall in Wiesbaden solely to hear Ehrlich. He gave a careful, scientific speech, but could not conceal the bombshell it contained, as he reported on the development of arsephenamine, better known thereafter as 606 or under the marketed name Salvarsan. Ehrlich was doing nothing less than introducing a miracle, a cure for syphilis. The applause was long and loud.

At subsequent medical conferences in 1910, Dr. Ehrlich needed a police escort just to make his way through the crowds that turned out to see him.[15] Thomas Edison called Ehrlich's discovery of Salvarsan one of the two great events of the year (the other being the prospect of a republic being formed in China).[16] *The New York Times* titled an article about Ehrlich's 1913 appearance at an international conference in London "World Doctors Hail Ehrlich as Hero."[17]

Beneath the applause, however, there were grumblings that Salvarsan was either ineffective or dangerous or both. Unfortunately, it had to be prepared for injection in a complicated procedure that required exact timing. Inadvertent errors in administering Salvarsan hurt its reputation in some circles. (An improvement, Neosalvarsan, was introduced in 1912; simpler and safer, it remained in use until 1943, when penicillin was recognized as an effective treatment for syphilis.)

During 1910–11, attacks against both Salvarsan and its discoverer escalated. The majority of doctors rejected charges that the drug was dangerous, but a small minority refused to let the issue rest. At the same time rumors swirled through the world press that Dr. Ehrlich was making vast profits from the sales, and had even purchased a new automobile for himself. That was the stuff of envy, probably stoked by anti-Semitism. Ehrlich supplied proof that he was donating his share of the profits to the Speyer Haus, to fund further research, and a colleague pointed out that the Ehrlichs were wealthy people who could have bought an automobile, if they wanted one, long before

606 came along. Most disturbing of all, some people implied that Ehrlich was trying to create a promiscuous society by offering a cure for syphilis.

The controversies, especially those within the scientific community, dismayed Dr. Ehrlich. In early 1911, he wrote to his friend Simon Flexner of the Rockefeller Institute in New York City, "The past year was a very hard one for me and I really feel how nervously exhausted I am. I must also say that I could have become old and have died without having had any notion of the meanness of mankind, which I now have had to experience."[18]

Perhaps it was fortunate that Dr. Ehrlich died in 1915, before he could experience the brunt of far greater human meanness and cruelty. Only sixty-one at the time of his final illness, he was exhausted from overwork—including, perhaps, the effort of smoking more than two dozen cigars a day. Dr. Paul Ehrlich had built one of the most productive careers in the history of German science, ending with fifteen years as the master of his own research compound in Frankfurt. The list of major honors accorded him runs to four pages of tight print in his biography. Yet when the Nazis came to power in 1933, they confiscated every available book about Ehrlich and burned it, as part of a campaign to destroy his name. Mrs. Ehrlich remained in Frankfurt with her two daughters and their husbands until 1938, when friends convinced them that they would be sent to the concentration camps if they stayed. Ehrlich's family emigrated to the U.S.

Dr. Ehrlich expanded every field he entered, including microbiology, serumology, and chemotherapy. That is what he left to the future of science. To future scientists, he left an example they couldn't follow, except by not following anyone: "He was always completely himself," recalled Carl Schleich, who knew him from their earliest days at the Charité Hospital in Berlin, "an original from top to toe; a man who had, absolutely, the courage of his almost absurd personality. For any student of character, he was living proof of the fact that true greatness has no need of pose, or concealment, or pretence."[19]

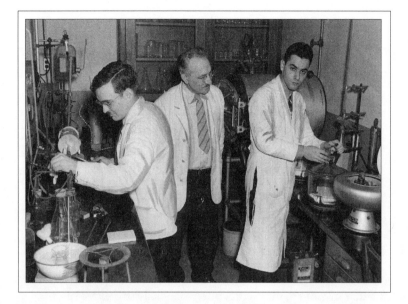

Dr. Selman Waksman and Albert Schatz
ET AL

For almost fifty years, the only regret surrounding the first known cure for tuberculosis was that not everyone connected with the discovery received due credit. It was a small-scale tragedy but a dramatic one, especially in view of the phenomenon created by the introduction of the new treatment, the drug streptomycin, in 1945. In the wake of that discovery, one man walked away with the gratitude of nations, a prominent place in scientific history, money and the chance to do something magnificent with it, and finally, a Nobel Prize: everything that a researcher dreams about as the long nights drag by in a laboratory. The other members of the team responsible for the discovery were left behind without much more than an interesting line to add to a résumé.

In truth, the name of the discoverer is the least important aspect of any medical breakthrough—the circumstances of the people helped by it matter more, and so does the reach of the ideas built upon it. Nonetheless, medical history has a unique ability to confer something like sainthood on those individuals who have presided over its high points. Their names are preserved along the longest unbroken continuum in Western civilization, the development of medical science. Immortality being fairly heady stuff and guarantees of it being truly rare, the drive for credit in an epochal medical discovery is itself a matter of life and death, or so it can appear to those in the hunt. The discovery of streptomycin made that clear and baffled so many of the people who stepped into the muddle created by it that, in the end, even the worker who washed out the test tubes was officially accorded some measure of the glory. But only Selman Waksman went home with the Nobel.

Waksman was born in Russia in 1888, in a town near Kiev. His family was, as he recalled, "a true matriarchate."[1] Its prosperity was due in large measure to his widowed grandmother's decision to go into business as a wholesale merchant. Though she had to be away from home most of every week, she made a good living, and Selman grew up in a comfortable setting, undoubtedly a mama's (and a grandmama's) boy. His father, a potmaker, didn't figure as prominently, living part of the time in another town. Because the Waksmans were Jewish, the educational opportunities open to Selman were limited. It required cunning for him just to slip through the official obstacles and graduate from high school. Originally, he thought he might go the University of Vienna to study medicine, but at about the time he was making his decision, his mother died. That changed the world he'd always known but it was his father's rather too hasty remarriage that ended it forever.

With nothing to stop him, Waksman sold his belongings and left Russia for America. He was one of 187,000 Russian immigrants to arrive in the U.S. in 1910.[2] However, there was nothing huddled, dazed or wide-eyed about Selman Waksman. As soon as he arrived, he applied for admission to Columbia University's College of Physicians and Surgeons and was accepted on the basis of his record in Russia. Still, because he was living with relatives in central New Jersey, he was also attracted to Rutgers University, where a professor in the Agricultural School spoke to him at length and argued that anyone who *really* wanted to pursue medical research would attend an agricultural college.[3] That may have been the kind of line that people handed recent immigrants in those days, but Waksman bought the idea and had no reason to regret it —especially since he couldn't afford the tuition at Columbia anyway. He entered Rutgers with the class of '15 and stayed there, in effect, for the rest of his life, taking his masters and doctorate and then becoming a professor.

Selman Waksman was justifiably pleased with himself, an immigrant who had risen to the top of his field in America. There was only one problem, and it rankled a person with Waksman's sense of pride: His chosen field was soil microbiology, and hardly anyone, even within the scientific community, knew what it was. With his trademark enthusiasm, Waksman set out to change that, writing dozens of articles to introduce the subject to the greater scientific community, ranging from 1925's "What Is Humus?"[4] to 1945's "Soil Microbiology as a Field of Science."[5] After twenty years, though, he had to admit that soil microbiology was still "only vaguely understood and often little appreciated."[6] It was an uphill battle, but then, that may have been what he liked about it.

One of Waksman's early articles was called "The Soil Population,"[7] a phrase that reflects the fascination of the field. Every pinch of dirt clinging to a boot or a horse's hoof teems with occupants in the form of bacteria, fungi, protozoa, algae, actinomycetes, and other plant and animal life invisible to the naked eye. It is tempting to call them "simple" forms of life, except that they aren't simple-looking, taking all kinds of shapes, and they especially aren't simple in their behavior. Soil microbiology is partly a soap opera, in which the individual microbes swirl around each other, deciding whether they are friends or competitors. It is also partly a brawl, because they waste no time killing their enemies. Sometimes they gobble each other up, but very often the weapon of choice is a chemical, produced by one microbe specifically to kill another. Looking through the microscope at soil samples all those years at Rutgers cannot have been dull for Selman Waksman.

However, neither Waksman nor the field of soil microbiology made any startling advances in the 1920s and most of the 1930s. Part of the reason was that, as Waksman himself wrote, there was always some question as to whether soil microbiology was more closely related to the biological sciences, including medicine, or the agricultural sciences, in the form of crop development. While that question played out, the field missed its early opportunities. In the early 1930s, for example, Dr. Waksman noticed that *Mycobacterium tuberculosis,* the microbe responsible for TB, thrived in soil that had been sterilized, yet was quickly destroyed in healthy, microbe-filled soil. Obviously, something (or someone) in the mix had the recipe for a TB-killing chemical. Waksman knew that much, yet he didn't pursue it. Soil microbiology, at that time, was just not aligned closely enough with medicine.

Meanwhile, other aspects of microbiology surged. In 1928, Professor Alexander Fleming of London discovered penicillin, a substance produced in a fungus that he just happened to find growing on a plate in his laboratory. Penicillin killed a number of virulent forms of bacteria, though the process for extracting it from the mold was imperfect and kept Fleming from announcing it as a medicinal drug. For the time being, it was exciting enough simply as proof that nothing could kill bacteria better than other bacteria.

Researchers in the 1930s were looking more and more carefully at microbes, trying to identify any that might become little arsenals for the benefit of mankind. As the leading soil microbiologist in the U.S., Dr. Waksman slowly woke up to the fact that his lab was perfectly positioned to take a position at the forefront, since it was already on familiar terms with thousands of microbes little known to other researchers. As Waksman liked to point out, the mold that alighted in Professor Fleming's lab and produced penicillin started out in the soil. It probably blew in through the window.

Between 1937 and 1941, Waksman started to shift his priorities away from agriculture and toward research into antibiotics—in fact, "antibiotic" was a term he coined himself in 1941. He defined it as "a chemical substance produced by a microbe which has the capacity to inhibit the growth of and even to destroy other microbes."[8]

After America entered World War II at the end of 1941, however, Rutgers University reset its priorities. It prepared to disband the department of soil microbiology and let Dr. Waksman go. Waksman was soon reprieved, in part because he stressed to administrators his new emphasis on identifying antibiotics for medical use. To that end, he oversaw a laboratory of about a dozen assistants and graduate students, working in an atmosphere of friendly chaos in a small, three-story building on the Rutgers campus. "Dr. Waksman is our great white father," said Doris Jones, a graduate student, during a speech much later in which she set the scene at the lab. "He is wise, demanding, yet understanding. He doesn't seem pretentious. His clothing is worn, and his vest always seems to carry traces of his last few meals, maybe a moth hole or two. He wants us to work hard, not waste lots of time studying extraneous things in books. I worship him."[9]

Waksman was universally admired by the members of his team, who worked with wide latitude on projects he managed from a distance. Two traits particularly endeared him to the students. First, he was always available for consultation and ready with expert advice. Second, he was unusually generous in sharing credit with his assistants on academic papers. Dr. Waksman encouraged female students to pursue graduate studies in microbiology; in his own listing of ten graduate students and researchers at the core of his antibiotic research, five were women.[10] One was Doris Jones, who worked in her own small lab in the basement. Another was Elizabeth Bugie, a graduate student. As her daughter, Eileen, explained, "My mom did a lot of work for Waksman. She was his lead technician, an extremely organized and meticulous person."[11]

In 1943, a former graduate student, Albert Schatz, joined the team, having recently been discharged from the Army because of a back problem. Dr. Waksman regarded him as unusually bright and had helped him to overcome financial problems in order to re-enroll at Rutgers as a graduate student. The two shared a common interest in finding an antibiotic that would destroy *Mycobacterium tuberculosis,* the well-fortified bacteria responsible for TB.

Waksman was motivated by a 1943 conference on TB that he

had attended in New York. After a discussion about the ability of common soil to kill *M. tuberculosis,* the general conclusion was that something in the excrement of earthworms must be responsible. While others went off to study worms, Waksman returned to Rutgers to look for the microbe that he felt was really responsible.

Schatz's interest in that same unidentified microbe came from a different direction. As of 1943, new developments in the study of penicillin had launched it into the news as a practically perfect antibiotic, able to destroy a wide variety of infections in the human body while causing nary a single side effect. However, one thing that penicillin could not do was kill the bacteria responsible for TB Schatz was particularly interested in finding an antibiotic to vanquish *M. tuberculosis.* Under Dr. Waksman's direction, he began to look for the answer among the actinomycetes.

For three and a half months, Schatz worked eighteen-hour days in his room in the basement of the Soil Microbiology building, finding samples and testing them for the ability to combat a whole group of disease-causing microbes, including *M. tuberculosis.* In addition to the cultures available at the lab, new samples came from scoopfuls of dirt, humus, and dust. The odds were steeply stacked against his isolating the one, or even ones, that he needed. But Albert Schatz was obsessed with the possibility.

One day an astute farmer in New Jersey heard one of his chickens wheezing. He rushed the bird to a state laboratory for testing, in fear that she was carrying an infectious disease. What she had, though, was a healthy crop of microbes growing in a film on her throat. After drawing samples on a swab, the pathologist at the lab identified them as actinomycetes and told the farmer the chicken was in no danger; she had probably just picked up the microbe pecking around in the ground for corn. The pathologist was aware that actinomycetes were Selman Waksman's specialty, and so he sent a culture to Rutgers, where Waksman recognized it as *Actinomyces griseus,* a microbe he and a colleague had discovered and named almost thirty years before. Waksman gave the culture to Doris Jones for use in a program of tests she was running. When Jones was finished with it, she suggested that Schatz might as well take it for his research. She passed it to him through a window between their two rooms in the lab. He ran it through his tests and several days later looked at the results.

"On October 19, 1943, at about 2 P.M.," Schatz later recalled, "I realized I had a new antibiotic. . .I sealed the test tube by heating the open end and twisting the soft, hot glass. . . I felt elated and very tired."[12]

Schatz knew the discovery was momentous, simply because it was an antibiotic, and he kept the first test tube of the microbe, which had been renamed *Streptomyces griseus,* to give to his mother (it is now in the collection of the Smithsonian Institution). He knew that it produced a chemical he called streptomycin. And he knew that streptomycin killed *M. tuberculosis*—or he thought he knew. Dr. Waksman immediately brought in other members of the research staff to extend the research into Schatz's discovery. Elizabeth Bugie was directed to verify his results. The short article introducing the promising antibiotic was published in *Science* in August 1944, authored by Doris Jones, H. J. Metzger, Albert Shatz, and Selman Waksman, in that order.[13] A more extensive piece appeared in December 1944, carrying the names of Schatz, Bugie, and Waksman.[14]

The question of credit for the discovery didn't much matter at the time the article came out, because the team at Rutgers had only seen streptomycin in action in petri dishes. They didn't know whether it would prove dangerous to a living person, and they didn't know how to manufacture it in usable quantities. Two research scientists at the Mayo Foundation volunteered to work on the first problem, and Merck Inc., the pharmaceutical company located in New Jersey, stepped in to help with the second. When Merck became involved, however, so did a battalion of lawyers, who made sure that streptomycin was patented, even if it was still untried. Schatz and Waksman were parties to the patent, but Bugie was not. In Waksman's opinion, the only reason to participate in a scientific patent was to boost one's career; since Bugie was planning to marry and stop working, he advised her not to press her case to join in the patent. She agreed, and expressed no regret over her decision in later years.

On November 20, 1944, streptomycin was administered to a human being for the first time, in a trial at the Mayo Clinic.[15] The patient, a 21-year-old woman, was suffering from tuberculosis and was in critical condition when the program began. After five months' worth of injections and two more years of rest, she was completely rid of TB. Obviously, streptomycin was no overnight miracle, but it could cure a disease that doctors had been able to coax and coerce but never before control. The U.S. Armed Forces placed an order for streptomycin in August 1945 and launched a massive trial program with it.[16]

By itself, streptomycin was found to be somewhat limited, due in part to the side effects, including ulcers, hair loss, and deafness, that it caused in some patients. With the introduction of companion drugs, however, its efficacy was increased to a very high level. Only four years after Schatz's discovery in October 1943, deaths due to TB had already started to fall notably. For the first time in history, TB was turned back, as an extract from a 1962 World Health Organization statistical chart shows.

Tuberculosis Morbidity and Mortality in Selected Countries[17]

Country	Death Rate: average annual rate per 100,000 population		
	1937-39	1947-49	1958
Canada	56.2	37.1	6.0
Chile	253.0	209.9	51.7
U.S.A.	50.0	29.9	7.1
England and Wales	63.8	49.4	9.9
Denmark	39.8	24.4	4.6
France	118.1	73.5	24.3

| Australia | 39.2 | 27.6 | 5.5 |
| Japan | 208.9 | 178.0 | 39.4 |

The success of streptomycin against TB came along like a gift in the wake of World War II—if nothing else, it was proof of the fresh start that science could give to the world. In the late 1940s and early 1950s, hundreds of articles were written each year about streptomycin. Selman Waksman was a constant center of attention, giving interviews and accepting invitations to lecture on streptomycin— and soil microbiology, when he could get that in. In the whirlwind, he spent more time in the laboratory than he ever had during the crucial years of 1943–44—but he was only giving tours to reporters and posing for pictures. In truth, his place had not been in the lab during the years of research; he was the leader who set the course and kept his team on it.

The publicity surrounding Waksman rankled Albert Schatz, who had originally felt as though they were partners in the discovery. "At first," Schatz recalled in 2002, "he'd invite me to his office to meet journalists, but after a while he stopped. I learned about what was going on, even the exciting developments at the Mayo Clinic, from magazines and newspapers. They were written by people who got all their information from Waksman. Eventually, he took full credit for the discovery."[18]

Having earned his doctorate, Schatz left Rutgers University abruptly in 1946, believing he was being slighted. However, he could at least content himself with the fact that the patent was being put to good use. The royalties that he and Waksman would have earned from streptomycin, estimated at $200,000 per month in 1949,[19] were to go into a trust to fund further research at Rutgers. With that understanding, Schatz went on to a teaching post at Brooklyn College, at $4,950 per year. Then he heard that Waksman had struck separate deals from which he was reaping substantial profits. That wasn't a fine point of ethics, it was a violation of the legal agreement between them. Schatz filed suit on March 10, 1950, claiming that he had been coerced into signing away his rights and demanding an accounting.[20] And as long as the topic had come up, thanks to Waksman's blunder, Schatz wanted much more than mere money—he wanted credit for his work.

A pretrial hearing revealed that Waksman had realized $350,000 in royalties before the funds were assigned to Rutgers. Within a few months, a New Jersey judge negotiated a settlement by which Dr. Waksman acknowledged that Albert Schatz was "entitled to credit legally and scientifically as codiscoverer of streptomycin."[21] If that and the stipulated $125,000 payment to Schatz had been the extent of the settlement, then streptomycin might be known to this day as a Waksman-Schatz discovery.

However, the judge also responded to Waksman's protest that Schatz had only been part of a larger team. "Streptomycin," said Waksman's lawyer before the trial, "is the result of nearly thirty years of continuous, systematized study by Dr. Waksman in the field of microbiology. Dr. Schatz was a graduate student under Dr. Waksman. He was one of about twenty graduate students and assistants who aided Dr. Waksman from time to time."[22]

As Waksman put it, more bluntly, Schatz was just lucky to be "in at the finish." The judge didn't forget all the others, taking half of Waksman's 20 percent royalty and dividing it among fifteen researchers, including Albert Schatz, who had worked under Waksman or with him in the development of the streptomycin discovery. Twelve more people connected with the discovery received lump sums. One of them was the widow of the man who had washed the test tubes and bottles in the lab.

More than two dozen people were to receive some compensation. As a legal maneuver, that aspect of the settlement was too effective to have been an accident of goodwill. Ever afterward, it would be hard to say specifically who had discovered streptomycin.

Waksman's lawyers traded a couple of percentage points in royalties (already assigned to Rutgers anyway) for a good chance at retaining full credit. "If you ask who was responsible for the isolation of the particular streptomycin-producing strain of *Streptomyces griseus*," Dr. Waksman wrote in his 1964 memoir of the discovery, "the answer must be that it was the chicken, because it was she who picked up the culture from the soil."[23] He wasn't just being facetious. Just as in the settlement, he was daring anyone who didn't buy his claim for sole credit to make a long, perhaps endless list of all the people, and chickens, who played a lesser part. Among those who chose not to try to compile such a list were the members of the Nobel committee who awarded the 1955 prize in Medicine and Physiology to Dr. Selman Waksman and no one else. Even after his nominal retirement three years laer, Waksman remained active in the field of microbiology. He died in 1973.

The ambiguity and sore feelings over the assignment of credit may have started with the articles produced by Waksman's lab during the first year of the discovery.[24] He very conspicuously listed various of his assistants as coauthors on each of them, even going so far as to bill their names above his. The typical research director wouldn't have made that gesture. Waksman probably wouldn't have done so, either, if he had to do it over. In a 1954 speech about the satisfaction of a career in research, he paused to make an reflection: "The question frequently arises of how to distribute the credit for a new discovery, a new fact, a new observation," he said. "Some investigators will credit their assistants merely by footnotes on scientific papers.

"Others," he continued, obviously referring to himself in the days of the streptomycin discovery, "will exert every effort to encourage their students, inspire them, and stimulate them further to select research careers, and in doing so, may not only add their names to the scientific papers but even place them first. In most cases, the results of the second practice are entirely satisfactory. Often, however, the consequences are most unexpected. How should one strike a happy medium? Scientists are searchers of truth. But they are also human beings."[25]

And if they have as much fight as any good *Streptomyces griseus*, they might also be immortals.

Thanks to streptomycin and the drugs that augmented it, most governments presumed that the battle against tuberculosis was practically won in the 1970s. Cutbacks in funding for campaigns against the disease were followed by complacency, with the result that in 1993, the World Health Organization had to take what it called "an unprecedented step," labeling the resurgence of TB a global emergency. By then, streptomycin was no longer the primary treatment for the disease, having been replaced by other drugs, but that was a moot point for health officials in the face of a threat from a mutant, drug-resistant strain of the TB bacillus. The situation has shown improvement since 1993. The rate of growth has slowed in most regions, but it would be a mistake to ever again regard progress as victory where tuberculosis is concerned.

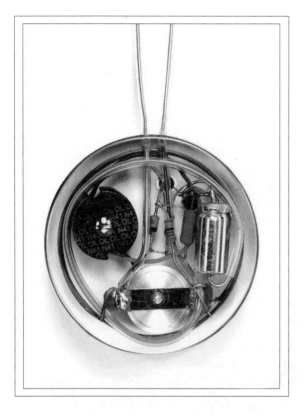

Arne and Else-Marie Larsson
BATTERY OPERATED

M edical history is typically told in terms of the doctors, the researchers, or even the outright crackpots who move it forward—and then go home at night. The patients they leave behind are less important, something like the members of an audience who benefit from a star turn but don't really affect it. In the case of the cardiac pacemaker, the electrical device that keeps millions of heart patients alive, the doctors had to share the glory with a battalion of engineers, but it wasn't any of them who actually started the revolution. The crucial push came in 1958 from a patient named Arne Larsson—and more specifically, from his wife, Else-Marie.

The Larssons lived in Stockholm with their two children. Arne, an electrical engineer, had been an amateur hockey player in the 1930s, playing for Sweden against teams from other nations. He was a tall man with broad shoulders and a strapping build, well-suited to sports. In the early 1940s, he settled down to a pleasant, quiet life with Else-Marie. Sweden was neutral during World War II, and so while most Europeans of Arne's age (he was born in 1915) had their lives interrupted if not ruined by the war, he lived the good life. And it showed: By 1952, Arne Larsson was a prosperous thirty-seven-year-old with an easy smile. Just four years later, he was a "cardiac cripple," according to a physician who knew him, "in a hopeless situation."[1]

Larsson just barely survived a bout with hepatitis in 1953, contracted from a plate of oysters, he ruefully maintained. An associated infection ravaged his heart and left it permanently scarred. As a result, his heart would beat at different rates, fast to slow. Sometimes it forgot, in effect, to beat at all. When that happened, Larsson fainted and had to be given a hard punch on the chest, which would make his heart pick up its beat. For a year or two, that was a way of life for Larsson, but in 1958, his condition worsened. He lay in a bed at the Karolinska Hospital in Stockholm, unable to walk more than four or five steps, and suffering up to thirty heart interruptions per day.

Larsson wasn't having heart attacks; for the most part, his heart and its functions, including the valves, the muscle tissue, and the overall blood flow, were perfectly fine. The scarring left by the infection had damaged only one small component, the sinus node, which is so small that it wasn't even discovered until 1907, after countless heart dissections over hundreds of years had missed it. The sinus node generates the rhythm of the heart and transmits it as an electrical impulse to the AV (atrioventricular) node, which delivers it to the rest of the heart. If either the sinus node or the AV node fails, then the heart will operate just like a broken clock: too fast, too slow, or not at all.

The effect of electricity on the heart had been known since the eighteenth century. In a storied incident from 1774, a little girl in London tumbled down a flight of stairs, causing her heart to stop. One of the doctors who rushed to the scene sent "electric pulses" into various parts of her body; when he finally attached his apparatus to her chest, right over the heart, her own pulse started up again and she made a complete recovery.[2] The same procedure failed to work in numerous other cases, though, probably because resuscitation can't occur unless the jolt of electricity is applied very soon after the heart has stopped. Doctors didn't know that then, but they did know that there was some relationship between electricity and heart activity.

Their imaginations ran wild. They fairly dashed to morgues to try electricity on cadavers, expecting them to spring to life. When that didn't succeed, they arranged to send impulses into the bodies of prisoners only minutes after the guillotine had struck, to see if the heart would revive. That didn't work, either. But if doctors could take electrical stimulation to its furthest conclusion, then so could authors, as Mary Wollstonecraft Shelley proved with her 1818 novel, *Frankenstein,* about a scientist who brings a corpse back to life. As frightening today as ever, it was written in the wake of the initial research into the relationship between electricity and the body.

Optimism soon turned to cynicism, though. Through much of the nineteenth century, the use of electricity as a medical tool was confined to a large and busy corner of the quack market. Unfortunately, it could be dangerous, as well as expensive. Because fakery abounded, honorable doctors tended to shy away from electricity as a medical treatment in the 1800s.

Scattered experiments in the early 1900s proved the worth of electrical equipment in monitoring the pulmonary system and in assisting it to some degree. In 1930, a doctor at New York University, A. S. Hyman, produced a machine that could deliver impulses to a heart that had stopped. It weighed sixteen pounds, had to be wound every six minutes, and was used only on rabbits.[3] Nonetheless, it was an early example of a cardiac pacemaker, and in spirit it was the ancestor of them all. Hyman's most important contribution of all was simply to give new respectability to therapeutic uses of electricity.

During World War II, Dr. Paul Zoll, an American doctor, was stationed at an Army hospital in England. He had been through Harvard Medical School, but he had never seen the heart as vividly as when he watched a colleague performing operations to remove shrapnel from the chests and even the beating hearts of wounded soldiers. "The heart appeared indeed to be a very sensitive organ that responded readily with ventricular contractions to stimuli," he later wrote.[4] Working at Boston's Beth Israel Hospital after the war, Zoll began to study electricity from an engineer's point of view.[5]

In 1952, he introduced the first pacemaker, or pulse generator, as it was sometimes called.

Zoll's machine gave doctors an important new tool. It was mainly used on patients whose hearts frequently stopped for lack of internal stimulus, a condition known as Stokes-Adams syndrome. Though it smoothed the rocky pace of the heartbeat in patients with Stokes-Adams, the drawbacks were many. The machine was so big it had to be pushed around on a cart. The wires carrying impulses from the machine were attached to the outside of the patient's chest, meaning that while the heart received a jolt, so did the muscles and bones in the upper chest. Moreover, that jolt had to be robust to make its way all the way through the flesh to the heart. It often left burns.

In most cases, a person would stay connected to the machine around the clock and when the heart stalled, the electrical impulses would begin, not ceasing until the heartbeat resumed on its own. Patients were undoubtedly grateful the first time the pulse generator saved the day, but over the course of weeks or months, the horrific pain that came with each treatment was more than many could bear.

Dr. Marcel Tuchman, who practiced medicine in New York City, saw many patients with Stokes-Adams, including an elderly woman he still remembered fifty years later. "When the heart stopped," he said, recalling the Zoll pulse generator, "an electric jolt was delivered to it and it started. But this happened twenty to thirty times in the course of the day. Now you can imagine this old lady with this terrible disease having to jerk in order to live—and there was no way that she could be separated from this device. Ultimately, she put a piece of cotton between the electrode and her chest wall and did not have that jolt delivered, and, as was expected, she died."[6]

Arne Larsson's bout with hepatitis had left him with a classic case of Stokes-Adams. By 1958, when his condition became critical, the external pulse generator was out of favor for people with chronic problems. It might be used to restore a heartbeat temporarily, but long-term cases were treated with drugs and other therapies, generally without success. None of them worked for Arne Larsson. He was a strong person, except for the tiny but terribly significant sinus node. Because it was failing, though, he was going to die. Stokes-Adams syndrome never ended in a miracle by itself. Quite the contrary: At some point, a patient just ran out of lucky breaks.

Else-Marie Larsson, informed by many doctors that Arne had only a short time left, refused to give up hope. She was especially determined that her husband would survive after she heard that one of the doctors at the Karolinska Hospital was working on a new kind of pacemaker, one that was implantable. With that, Mrs. Larsson made it her business to find the doctor, Åke Senning, and speak to him. Meanwhile, Arne was preparing himself for death.

"His wife begged us to try and help him by implanting our new pacemaker system," Dr. Senning later wrote.[7]

Arne Larsson, though confined to his bed, was fully aware of what was going on. "My wife attacked the doctor night and day," he recalled, "She said, 'Doctors, you must do something.' "[8]

"I said 'Please, please, you must try!' " Else-Marie recalled, concerning her conversations with Dr. Senning, " 'You must do it!' And then after a while, he said, 'I will talk with Dr. Elmqvist and we will come back to you.' "[9]

Rune Elmqvist, then fifty-two, was a medical doctor, but one who had never actually practiced. Instead, he had become a medical engineer, working with electrocardiograph machines and a rudimentary defibrillator. Since 1957, Elmqvist had been working with Senning to develop an implantable pacemaker. His first reaction to Else-Marie Larsson's plea was that the pacemaker under development was simply not ready for a human test. Senning was more inclined to see Else-Marie's point of view—perhaps in part because he was exactly Arne's age. From close up, forty-three probably seemed much too young to die.

Senning was a surgeon, but he knew firsthand about electricity and its effect on the heart:

My first experience with cardiac arrhythmia [momentary stoppage] was unforgettable. I had built a radio with a double-grid vacuum tube in the amplifier, and by chance I was able to hear Lindbergh's landing in his *Spirit of St. Louis* in Paris in 1927. My father translated to me what was happening. Shortly afterwards, while doing my schoolwork, I noticed a buzz in the radio each time I touched the iron lamp on my table. Once I grabbed the ground wire with the other hand. The effect was sensational. The lamp fell on the floor and I had a feeling my heart had stopped for a long time. The 220 volts of AC current from the lamp had probably caused a short period of ventricular fibrillation.[10]

Electricity could overwhelm the heart's own electrical system, as in Senning's boyhood experience, or restore it. The latter possibility drew Dr. Senning back to electricity, at a safe distance, during the early 1950s, when he was a familiar face at high-level cardiology conferences around the world. In 1954, he made a tour of the U.S. to visit researchers at the forefront of cardiac mechanization in its various forms. His first stop was Philadelphia, where Dr. John Gibbon worked, "to see the American state of the art," as he said.[11] Dr. Senning was aware of every important advance and returned from a 1957 tour of the U.S. particularly impressed, certain that he had seen "the beginning of the era of clinical pacing."[12] What he had seen, while observing Dr. Walt Lillehei at the University of Minnesota Medical School, was a new method of stitching electrodes directly to the heart, as opposed to the Zoll technique of attaching them to the outer wall of the chest.

Senning realized that if the electrodes were going to be attached directly to the heart, the battery and generator should follow. The whole pulse-generating apparatus belonged within the body. Of course, that wasn't likely to happen when the equipment was as big as a tea cart, but Senning had his brainstorm in the first blush of the transistor age. The work of a whole row of vacuum tubes could be accomplished by a single transistor, as small as a thumbnail and almost as flat.

Upon returning to Stockholm, Senning formed an alliance with an electronics firm, Elema-Schonander. Elmqvist, a senior engineer at the firm, eagerly followed Senning's initiative and set to work solving the many problems presented by the creation of an implantable pacemaker. A more resourceful man probably could not have been found.[13] Senning was lucky, and so was Arne Larsson.

Senning and Elmqvist had been at work for less than a year when Else-Marie Larsson began to implore them to use the new device to save her husband. Elmqvist argued against it, saying that animal testing had only just begun and that the future of the project would only be jeopardized by a premature human trial. Still, Arne Larsson was a rare candidate for a new device, being a fairly young person who was physically strong, except for the fact that his heart wouldn't work. Purely from the research point of view Senning and Elmqvist couldn't be sure when they would see another volunteer so well suited to their purposes.

The decision to go ahead with the surgery rested with Dr. Senning. No doubt he was influenced by Else-Marie's well-orchestrated campaign. As a friend once said, "Those who know Else-Marie Larsson recognize her as very persuasive."[14] The operation was scheduled for October 8, 1958. In theoretical terms, Elmqvist was ready. However, the only pacemakers he had on hand were meant for dogs. Working at home in his kitchen, he built the human version of the first implantable pacemaker. Then he made a spare. "Dr. Elmqvist rigged up circuits for two pacemakers," Senning recalled, "and molded them in epoxy resin in a shoe wax can measuring 55 mm [2 ⅛ inches] in diameter and 15 mm [a half-inch] in height."[15]

In the operating room, Åke Senning connected two stainless steel electrodes to Larsson's heart and nestled the shoe wax can containing the pacemaker into a fleshy part of Larsson's lower back. The operation went well and Larsson had his first good day in two years, with the pacemaker signaling his heart to beat at a steady 70 beats per minute. Recalled Else-Marie, "I went home about twelve o'clock in the night, and at two o'clock I phoned the hospital. And the nurse told me when I said who I was, 'Mrs. Larsson, I will ask for Dr. Senning.' And then, when you get that answer, you already know that something is wrong."[16]

The pacemaker had quit. But the next morning, Senning implanted a replacement, and it lasted for almost a year. Senning and Elmqvist made subsequent improvements to their technology, and the Elema 135 pacemaker went on the market in 1959. Two were sold that year. It was a start, albeit a small one.

Even Elmqvist was uncertain about the future of heart gadgetry. "I must admit that I had regarded the pacemaker more or less as a technical curiosity," he later wrote.[17] Others regarded the pacemaker as an immoral encroachment on the sanctity of the human body, reducing the very miracle of life to a series of blips and twitters emanating from a little box. "Many people," recalled Paul Zoll, "including my own cardiac fellow, thought it might be blasphemous, improper or unethical to keep a patient alive by such artificial means."[18] Patients themselves frequently voiced religious concerns over the implantation of a pacemaker.

"We were more realistic," Else-Marie Larsson reflected, "about how thin the thread is between life and death."[19]

For more than forty years, Arne Larsson's life served as a reply to any concerns that the heavens might disapprove of a pacemaker. Because of the device and further treatment, he wasn't reaching the end of his life in 1958—he was only halfway through it. He returned to work and became the head of a consortium of Swedish engineering firms in the mid-1960s. Six months out of each year, he traveled to exotic locales—by himself, with no one to punch his chest—overseeing shipboard electrical systems. Genial and enthusiastic by nature, Larsson was obviously in good health.

Åke Senning moved to Switzerland in 1961 to accept a teaching position at the University of Zurich where he spent the rest of his career. Rune Elmqvist stayed in Sweden and remained active in the development of pacemakers and other electronic medical devices.

The major problem with the early pacemakers was the battery life, which was normally counted in months. Because of that, they were used on a limited basis during the 1960s. But the introduction of the lithium battery in 1972 was a watershed for pacemakers; under lithium power they hummed along for eight years, on average. Even as more sophisticated pacemakers were developed, spawning a new specialty within the field of cardiology, Arne Larsson grew into the role of ambassador, a man who could speak from experience, having had 26 pacemakers in all. He died in 2001 of skin cancer, but left a unique legacy for millions of patients to follow.

"I forget I have a pacemaker," he once said in an interview, "because I have so much to do."[20]

IV
THE MIND

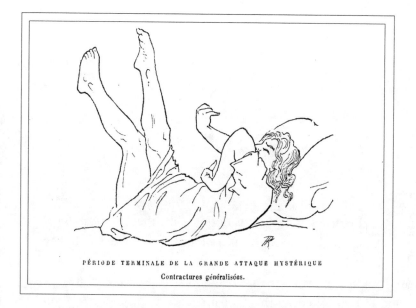

PÉRIODE TERMINALE DE LA GRANDE ATTAQUE HYSTÉRIQUE
Contractures généralisées.

Thomas Willis
ORGANIZED BRAIN

T he English Civil War was nothing like the American Civil War, which was a regional conflict, north versus south. The lines in the English war didn't start on a map. They appeared with the opinions that neighbors formed on white-hot issues: the amount of power that Parliament should wield in relation to that of the king, for instance, or whether a Protestant country like Britain should tolerate Catholicism. The men who left their homes to fill the ranks when the war broke out in 1642 were not professional soldiers by any means. In many of the battles, they tied sashes around their waists in lieu of uniforms—yellow for the Royalists and red for the opposition, known as Parliamentarians or Puritans.

One of the men who tied on the yellow sash for the king was Thomas Willis, a student about to graduate from Oxford University in 1642. Although most cities, including London, wavered in support of the differing sides during the war, Oxford was a stronghold for King Charles I, first to last. So was the Willis family. While the Civil War dragged on through the rest of the decade, Charles I spent several years living in the safe haven of Oxford, where he participated in futile negotiations with Oliver Cromwell, one of the Puritan leaders. By 1646, Cromwell was largely in control, impatient to yank England out of its ancient monarchy and transform it into a commonwealth. In 1649, Charles I was beheaded.

Thomas Willis had chosen the losing side in the war. Moreover, he lived in a city that was high on Cromwell's list of places to reform in the Puritan image. And worst of all, he defied Cromwell's most basic directives as soon as the Commonwealth began. By any normal standard, he should have felt the brunt of retaliation; at the very least, he should have grown destitute under a government he despised.

Quite the opposite. Very few people benefited more than Thomas Willis from the Cromwell years. He might have sincerely wished that Charles I had won the war and defended the status quo in English society. If that had happened, though, Willis probably couldn't have conducted the investigation of brain anatomy that was to make his reputation. He might not have left a foundation for the study of neurology and almost certainly couldn't have given the medical world its first constructive interpretation of brain disorders and mental illness, taking them at long last out of the realm of the unknown.

Willis's exploration of the brain was also radical as a major research project, in the modern sense of the term. Not only did it require sophisticated equipment, it relied on a spirit of teamwork new for the time. Moreover, the research confronted spiritual issues. For Thomas Willis to cross the divide between science and religion, and establish neurology in medicine, he would have to live through at least a couple of revolutions, in a historical zigzag he could use to his advantage. Fortunately, that is just what he got when his side lost the war.

Thomas Willis was born in 1621, in the town of Great Bedwyn in the rustic county of Wiltshire, west of London. His mother, Rachel, died when Thomas was ten. That is not much to go by, but at least it is definite. His father, also named Thomas, was either a butler or a farmer and may have attended Oxford University. Almost nothing about him is certain. The family could not have been very rich, though, because when Thomas the younger matriculated at Oxford, he was not listed as a gentleman or even as a paying commoner, but rather as a "batler," a lower-class student who had to work his way through school. Willis was fortunate in being assigned to attend a kindly school official named Dr.

Thomas Iles. It was Mrs. Iles who influenced him most, however, and probably inspired him to become a physician.[1]

John Aubrey, an Oxonian only five years younger than Willis, described the situation. Willis, he wrote, "was first servitor to Dr. Iles, one of the canons of Christ Church, whose wife was a knowing woman in physic and surgery, and did many cures. Tom Willis then wore a blue livery cloak and studied at the lower end of the hall, by the hall dore; was pretty handy, and his mistresse would oftentimes have him to assist her in making of medicines. This did him no hurt."[2] Mrs. Iles was part of a movement in healing called iatro-chemistry, which looked to chemical compounds rather than herbal remedies as prescriptions for specific complaints. Early iatrochemists were dismissed as mystics, looking for an elixir of life just as alchemists looked for a way to transform rocks into gold, but by the seventeenth century, iatrochemists were serious scientists, laying the foundation for pharmacology. Thomas Willis would be a committed iatrochemist,[3] studying symptoms and trying to match them with recognizable chemicals.

Learning chemistry with Mrs. Iles may have been the most exciting part of Willis's early undergraduate years. In school, his education was much more traditional—or even medieval, in the opinion of his biographer, Hansruedi Isler. The Oxford course then was strictly proscribed, relying on Latin and Aristotelian logic to train young minds and classes in general subjects to fill them: grammar, rhetoric, moral philosophy, geometry, astronomy, meta-physics, and music.[4] It was book-learning, from a shelf of very old books, and did little to inspire originality. Some of the students couldn't bear the drudgery, but Willis applied himself and was scheduled to graduate in June 1642.

That year, Charles I's desperate need for money forced him to recognize Parliament, which he did—in his own way. He decided to pay a personal visit to the House of Commons, something no monarch had ever done before, to arrest five of its least cooperative leaders. By the time he arrived with his warrant, however, the birds had flown, as he put it. Outmaneuvered, Charles left London and with that, each side readied for war. By the end of 1642, Charles had established his headquarters at Oxford University's Christ Church College, where Willis was a student. The king's physician, William Harvey, was also there. Willis's father had volunteered as a soldier in the Royalist army and Thomas was also involved with the cause, although he continued his studies and managed to earn his degree on time. In 1643, his father died of a fever while in camp with the army. Willis joined the university volunteer corps, training as an archer. Even while remaining a reserve soldier, he soon returned to school. Over the next three years, he attended medical school at the university, but in the summer of 1646, his soldiering days were through for good, as the king fled to Scotland. Willis received his medical degree that December and started his career in a country without a king, controlled by a Parliament that was itself controlled by small landowners and Puritans. Almost as soon as Charles left Oxford, the newfound power of Parliament descended upon it. The leading Royalists on the faculty were dismissed and disgraced. Dr. Iles, Willis's former employer, was among them. He would die in poverty in 1649.

The Puritans were maniacal on the topic of religious ceremony, which they believed should be minimal, and church finery, which they felt should be nonexistent. They also rejected hierarchy in the clergy. All were facets of the Anglican Church, which the Puritans believed leaned too far toward "popery," or Roman Catholic ways. Thomas Willis almost certainly took an obligatory oath of allegiance to the Parliament, but at the same time, he hosted Anglican church services in his home—which was patently illegal.

One might think that the Puritans, who were so rigid on churchly matters, would in due course squelch the intellectual life of the college. But alongside their conservative religious values was a vibrant interest in making money. In that spirit, the Puritans replaced Royalist professors with scientists of a more practical bent. Instead of being forced to look in crumbling books, the students were encouraged to make experiments—in the new atmosphere, knowledge was not merely to be memorized but extended. The very active practical scientists attached to Oxford "gave themselves the name of Vertuosi," wrote Anthony à Wood, who was at the university at the time, "and pretended to go beyond all others in the University for knowledge, which caused envy in many." Thomas Willis, the avowed Royalist and secret Anglican, was irresistibly drawn to the new professors. They may have been sent by the enemy, but they were going about things in a way that placed the future of science in the hands of the living and not the dead.

When Willis graduated from medical school, he was penniless. He could only afford a half of a horse, splitting the cost of one with another doctor. Willis was a good physician, though, and certainly a hardworking one. He was willing to travel further into the countryside than other Oxford physicians, and even learned to sleep on horseback to make better use of his long hours on the road. Within a few years, he built up a viable practice. During the late 1640s, Willis began to work in anatomical research at Oxford University on an informal basis. In 1650, he and another physician there received permission to dissect the body of a young woman condemned to hang. The woman, Anne Green, had been a maid in a country estate, where she was apparently raped by someone in the squire's family. Pregnant, she either had an abortion or killed her newborn baby; when she was found out, she received the death penalty.

On the appointed day, the noose was tightened around her neck and a ladder kicked out from under her feet. For several long moments, she hung, all right, but while her many friends looked on, she looked right back. She seemed to be dying a slow death, instead of a humanely quick one, and so her friends grabbed her feet and pulled down, even remaining suspended with her. They tugged from every angle, to put her out of her pain, until at last, it was over—anyway, the under-sheriff said that if they pulled any more, the rope might break. And so her body was put into a coffin and sent to Dr. Willis's rooms.

Willis and his colleague, Dr. William Petty, opened the box and noticed immediately that Anne Green's body was rattling. Upon investigation, they realized that she was still alive, breathing through a passageway that was damaged, understandably. "A young man standing by thought to put her out of her misery by stamping on her," according to a contemporary account.[5] Instead, Willis and Petty revived her with a little bloodletting and a dose of strong liquor. She became a ward of the medical college for a short time, until Willis and the others contributed to a dowry and found a decent man for her to marry. The outcome was only a little less fortunate for Willis than for the woman; he was famous around Oxford ever after as the doctor in the Anne Green case.

Thomas Willis was a man of average height, with a long face, high forehead, linear nose, and pointed chin. Wood described him as "a plain man, a man of no carriage, little discourse, complaisance, or society."[6] According to John Aubrey, Willis stammered. Willis's fortunes had risen with the overall prosperity of the middle class during the Commonwealth. In 1657, he married the sister of one of the priests giving services at his house; they would eventually have eight children, though only the eldest son survived to adulthood.

Due to his Royalist reputation, Willis couldn't join the faculty of Oxford, although he did continue to work closely with the new generation there.[7] The atmosphere of the school under the Commonwealth encouraged the spirit of actual *common-wealth,* or sharing, which was reflected in the teamwork with which projects were undertaken. Formerly, the best minds in science worked independently, with assistants but rarely with colleagues. The practical spirit of the Commonwealth encouraged the idea that bigger problems required more minds, working in cooperation. Willis, who had a natural ability to give and receive loyalty, was well suited to the new approach.

In 1658, Oliver Cromwell died of natural causes, leaving behind a checkered legacy of tolerance and slaughter, democracy, and, finally, dictatorship. His son Richard Cromwell ruled briefly, but the

Restoration saw Charles II accede to the throne in a peaceful transition in 1660. That same year, in the first wave of favors handed out to reward stalwart Royalists, Thomas Willis was named to the prestigious post of Sedleian Professor of Natural Philosophy at Oxford.[8] His assignment was to lecture on matters pertinent to the soul, and those who secured his appointment assumed that he would revert to the teachings of Aristotle.[9] It was too late for that, however.

Willis used his position to begin an ambitious new project, the most well-planned research project in the history of Western medicine to that point. Other people had certainly amassed huge bodies of work in previous years: Vesalius had surveyed human anatomy on a truly awesome scale; Harvey had studied the heart and blood vessels across a wide array of species. But Willis turned a new corner by encompassing other scientists in his work, drawing on the theme of commonwealth by sharing work and ideas, in addition to a final goal. That goal was to dissect the brain, relying on observation rather than previously published research. "Thomas Willis," wrote William F. Bynum, "applied the anatomical method to a system with functions not so easily elucidated as those of the circulatory or musculo-skeletal system."[10]

The men Willis drew around him were Christopher Wren, Thomas Millington, and Richard Lower. Lower was, in Willis's words, "a doctor of outstanding learning and an anatomist of supreme skill." He acted as the first assistant, who translated Willis's theories into investigations that could generate proof. Millington, a young doctor who would soon be engaged as physician in the court of Charles II, had already gained attention for his studies on plant reproduction. He would be Willis's successor as Sedleian Professor. Wren, accomplished in so many fields that an acquaintance called him "that miracle of a youth," was an expert microscopist for the time and analyzed brain tissue under the glass. He also provided drawings of the research findings. With colleagues of that caliber, there was not much that Willis couldn't accomplish. When the four met, Willis would typically direct Lower's dissections, while Wren and Millington added to the discussion or performed specialized research. The team seems to have developed a means, novel for the time, of preserving brain tissue, so that they could return to certain aspects of a dissection over the course of time. Another technique originated for the research involved the injection of ink into tissue for the sake of tracing patterns of fluid movement within the brain.

In previous dissections, anatomists would cut the skull in order to look at the brain from various angles. One of Willis's fundamental innovations was to remove the brain intact through the bottom of the skull.[11] Through that means, he couldn't help but make new observations. Under his direction, Lower conducted the most careful investigation up to that time of the cranial nerves, which connect parts of the face and upper chest directly to the brain. Willis identified nine pairs, though more modern research eventually identified twelve pairs. He correctly surmised the purpose of most of those he listed.[12] Willis's name was attached to the ring of arteries he described at the base of the brain. Though the vessels had been discovered a few years earlier by a German anatomist (Johann Wepfer), they became known in English medical circles as "the circle of Willis."[13]

In 1663, Willis requested permission from the government to publish his research in a book to be called *Cerebri Anatome* ("Anatomy of the Brain"), with drawings contributed by Wren and Lower. Under the Commonwealth, scientific research of almost any kind was granted a license for publication; but under Charles II, censorship was much more heavy-handed. *Cerebri Anatome* was a remarkably cogent and precise work, but it had to offer more than that to be published in Charles II's reign. It needed to convey a religious humility, and that was not necessarily easy to achieve when reaching into the mysteries of the mind. However, Willis, the Royalist who enjoyed the Commonwealth, was just the man to find a way.

Throughout his writings, Willis confirmed his belief that the soul had a physiological basis—that it actually resided in bodily matter.

Later researchers, including Franz Joseph Gall, would separate the mind from the soul and look only for evidence of the mind, in fact or function, within the brain.[14] Willis, however, was taking the longest step possible for a person in the mid-seventeenth century: attaching some physiological basis to the thoughts and feelings of mankind, all of which he was very quick to identify as subjects of the soul. Or souls: The innovation in his thinking lay in dividing the concept of the soul into three entities, one of which he assumed for science—the new science he termed neurology.

The soul that invited observation and even speculation, according to Willis, was the "sensitive" soul, which was common to all animal species, in his assertion. It was responsible for reflex, sensory perception, and movement. The other two souls retained a sense of spiritual mystery. The "rational soul" was the special province of humans, containing loftier characteristics such as force of will and reasoning; it was also the immortal soul. The "vital" soul, the most basic form of life-spirit, was contained somewhere in the body. Willis was not prepared to speculate on that (Harvey thought it resided in the blood), except to assert that it was also to be found in animals.[15]

While the explanation of the three souls was not acceptable to everyone, it did allow Willis to explore the brain to the extent of the sensitive soul. In the books that followed the publication of *Cerebri Anatome* in 1664, he described the brain in terms of pathology and comparative anatomy. Willis's work is at its best in describing brain anatomy, which it raises to a level of precision that did indeed establish neurology as a science grounded in fact and ripe with potential. In a second respect, Willis's books had an even wider influence, though.

The definition of the sensitive soul allowed Willis to speculate on the nature of illness in the brain, a topic that had previously been dominated by religious doctrine. When a person suffered from mental or nervous disorders, the cause was typically ascribed to the devil or the presence of sin in the person or the family. Willis used his theory of the two souls within the brain to suggest that one of them could be ill or damaged. In that way, he connected such problems as palsy, somnolence, nightmares, and headaches to physiological sources within the brain.[16] He was especially influential in his interpretation of epilepsy, a disorder that was previously misunderstood, as fits were often believed to reflect some sort of demonic possession. Admitting that he was using a word new to medicine, Willis described an epileptic fit as a kind of "explosion" within the brain itself.[17] He went on to accurately describe various kinds of seizures and attribute them to the nervous system.

Thomas Willis gave neurology a starting point. Though *Cerebri Anatome* contained flaws, it also carried a sense of purpose that has made it a frame of reference for research into the brain ever since.

Willis did not forsake his medical practice while he was directing the research on the brain. In fact, his earnings as a physician made him the highest-paid man in Oxford—he took home about £300 per year, at a time when a cook at the university, for example, earned £2 per year.[18] His trick was quite simple: He attracted rich clients and charged them outrageous fees—which they paid willingly. Not only was Willis a fine diagnostician, he had a long list of remedies that he had devised over the years. To keep them secret, he employed his own apothecary.

In times that rewarded expedience, Thomas Willis, the man who could sleep on horseback, never wasted a minute. He died of pneumonia in 1675, at the age of fifty-four.

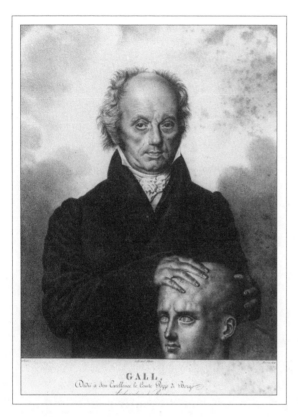

GALL,
Dédié à son Excellence le Comte Rizzo di Marco

Franz Joseph Gall
LOST IN THOUGHT

At state fairs and along boardwalks, a few phrenologists still ply the old trade, examining head structure and producing a personality report based on the findings. As a business, though, phrenology is barely a whisper of what it was in the 1840s, when it commanded excited crowds in palatial establishments in every American city. Occupying old mansions or new downtown buildings, phrenology "museums" offered displays, readings, and lectures. They also had shops, with shelves full of the accoutrements: "books, busts, charts, skulls—every requisite for the study of this interesting science," as an advertisement in Charleston, South Carolina, expressed it.[1]

Astrology, palm reading and handwriting analysis have long since surpassed phrenology, even on the carnival fringe of society, where people flock to find out who they are, in suitably small dollops of information. Perhaps any process that promises to reveal a person's innermost characteristics can have commercial appeal, at least for a while. No matter what the specific results happen to be, though, they all carry the same reassurance: that personality is inborn.

Now medicine is close to proving the same thing. The nascent field of brain mapping is intent on using physical facts to nail down personality, that most ephemeral of human possessions. Genes responsible for everything from thrill-seeking to nervousness to the propensity to marry a rich person are being identified across large population groups and even traced to particular parts of the brain. One of the most advanced programs is the Brain Mapping Division at the School of Medicine at the University of California at Los Angeles. In 2002, three scientists working there made a striking announcement in the *Annals of Medicine:* "We recently developed a large-scale computational brain atlas," they wrote, "to store information on individual variations in brain structure and their inheritability."[2]

Franz Joseph Gall could have made much the same statement, two hundred years earlier. As the physician who originated phrenology, he created a brain atlas, too. The tools at his command were a far cry from the mainframe computers and magnetic resonance imaging machines used at UCLA and in dozens of other brain-mapping projects around the world. Nonetheless, Gall did remarkably well, not because his map was accurate but because he succeeded in promoting the idea that the functions of the brain actually emerge from a spatial organization—that the brain does indeed have a map. Before Gall, the brain was usually regarded as a generalized cloud of matter, and certainly no one would bother making a map of a cloud. Some powerful people, including Napoleon Bonaparte, believed it should stay that way, in a kind of cloud of useful uncertainty. The old sense of order in society was dependent on it, or so they thought.

Franz Joseph Gall was born in Germany of Italian descent.[3] His parents, though hardly rich (his father was a small-time merchant), provided him with a good education locally, but in 1781, he left for Vienna, where he graduated from medical school four years later. Angular in build, Gall was a distinctly intelligent-looking man, not because of his high forehead, framed by rings of wavy hair, nor because of the fine features of his face, but rather because of his eyes. In his portraits, at least, they are intent and tinged with impatience.

As a doctor in Vienna, Gall established a thriving practice but continued to study in his spare time, becoming a skilled anatomist. He was especially expert in the way he treated the brain, which tended to present a puzzle for anyone who was attracted to the mechanical beauty in the other organs: the heart as a pump, the kidney as a filter, the lungs as a bellows. The brain had all the beauty of a cauliflower and was just about as mechanical. Little more than that was likely to be learned, given the way that anatomists typically attacked it. Dr. Gall made his reputation in 1790s with a new method he devised for cutting the brain very deftly, in order to display at least some of its interconnecting nerves.[4] Even one of his later adversaries, Pierre Flourens, recalled at a distance of fifty years, "I shall never forget the feeling I experienced the first time I saw Gall dissect a brain. It seemed to me that I had never seen this organ before."[5] Even if Gall had never developed his theories on the workings of the brain, his reputation in neuroscience would rest securely on his early observations in brain anatomy. Indeed, they gave him the prominence to offer a radical new theory at the close of the eighteenth century.

In studying the brain, Gall could not help trying to understand it as a machine, something like the other organs in the body. To do that, though, he had to cross over a line that separated medicine from religion. And another separating medicine from philosophy. And another separating medicine from government. Gall was not the first person to consider the functions of thought and feeling in physiological terms, but he arrived with better preparation than anyone else had. With his theory, he intended to address the relationship between the brain—the rightful domain of doctors—and the mind, which had long been the province of religion, philosophy, and government.

Gall began developing his ideas in 1792 and lecturing on them in 1796. At that time, the prevailing theory was that the brain operated as the center of immediate mental processes, including, for example, sensation and reflex, but that the greater part of the mind, including all of the factors of personality that differentiate one person from another, were dictated by the soul. In some languages, there were not even two different words for "mind" and "soul." They were reckoned to be the same thing.

Anyone who believed that the mind was merely a reflection of earthbound factors was regarded, often with contempt, as a materialist. In the eighteenth century, a materialist was not a person who wanted lots of shoes, but rather someone who denied the influence of the gods over anything except the general scheme of life itself. A materialist sat at the opposite end of the spectrum from a spiritualist, who thought that each person was a constant reflection of heavenly intervention. The spiritualist presumption of the time was that by and large people were born in the circumstances in which they belonged. Therein lay order in society.

The spiritualist position suited most of those responsible for (or benefiting from) stability in the late 1700s, notably monarchs and the nobility. Most doctors, for their part, steered clear of any controversy on the topic. The accepted way to discuss personality, for example, was in terms of "physiognomy," which studied the imprint of the mind on the face. Johann Lavater, a minister from Switzerland, wrote a veritable best-seller on the subject in 1787, explaining in detail how the face betrayed the hidden secrets of character. According to his teachings, people could never overcome the faces or, concomitantly, the souls with which they were born. The theory slid naturally into a discussion of ideal beauty, and from there into outright racism.[6] Physiognomy, however, remained within the bounds of acceptability in European societies, because it didn't suggest where the various aspects of personality came from, only how they could be detected.

As Gall hovered over his anatomical table in the 1790s, exploring the brain and trying to understand it, he couldn't help recalling that when he was a boy in Germany, he'd noticed that among his classmates, those with similar skull structure also had similar personality traits. He particularly remembered noting that the students who had the best memories had eyes that bugged out. Anyone with a clear recollection of junior high school knows what he meant. As an anatomist, Gall was compelled to make a connection between those bugging eyes and a large capacity for memory; his conclusion was that the part of the brain containing memory must be at the front—near the eyes, as a matter of fact. The more memory, the less room within the skull for deep-set eyes.

Gall made extensive observations of people in Vienna, paying special attention to criminals and others with exaggerated personality traits. He had help from several assistants, most prominently a fellow German named Johann Spurzheim. A medical school student, Spurzheim was eighteen years younger than Gall, though the two would eventually work as collaborators.

The basis of the theory that Gall christened "organology" was that the brain was composed of many separate but cooperative organs. Each was responsible for some aspect of the personality; the more prominent the organ, the more pronounced the trait. The head shape was not by itself crucial to the personality. However, the skull was presumed to adapt to the shape of the various organs within the brain. Therefore, the shape of the skull denoted the structure of the brain and, according to Gall, the mind within. Though Gall's method was later derided as "bump-ology" or "skull-juggling," he was, in fact, studying the living brain in the only way available to him: by looking at the shape of the head. Where modern researchers make brain scans, he took plaster casts. Among his subjects were hundreds of criminals and at least a few people celebrated for their intellectual powers.

By 1802, Dr. Gall's lectures in Vienna were less likely to feature a dissection of the brain than a surprisingly precise description of the function of the organs within it. With all of the authority at his command, he told audiences that the collection of organs in the brain reflected the unity of the mind and body. That directly contradicted a widely accepted belief called dualism, which held that the two were separate: that the beautiful abstraction of the mind was naturally separate from the tired junkheap of the body. For the conservative city of Vienna, it was something of a thrill to hear such an eminent scientist express such radical ideas. While people continued to crowd into the lectures in 1798, Gall composed an open letter in which he announced his plan to publish a complete description of the functions of the brain.

With that, the Austrian royal family had had enough of Dr. Franz Joseph Gall. All over Europe, in fact, conservatives and monarchists were suspicious that organology would give people the impression that nothing in the human experience—including the divine right of kings—was preordained by God.[7] "This doctrine concerning the head," wrote Emperor Francis I in 1801, "which is talked about with enthusiasm, will perhaps cause a few to lose their heads."

"It leads to materialism," His Highness added, "therefore [it] is opposed to the first principles of morals and religion."[8] Francis I ordered Gall to stop giving his lectures, and revoked his right to publish any books in Austria. Gall wasn't in fear for his life, but he did have to make an immediate decision regarding his future. At forty-four, he could remain in Vienna, a respected and prosperous physician. Or he could leave and start over somewhere, for the sake of his controversial theory.

Whatever the contours of his own head, Gall had a vivid personality in several respects. He particularly loved science, gardening, and money. He also loved the company of women, though not always that of his wife.[9] In part because his domestic life was so strained, Gall felt no remorse in leaving Vienna; his only regret was having to abandon his garden. For the next two years, he had no permanent home, but roamed Northern Europe on a triumphant lecture tour, in the company of Johann Spurzheim. Though Spurzheim would eventually shine as the more effective promoter of the two, Gall undoubtedly had his own way with public opinion. By 1807, when he arrived in Paris, he was a bona fide celebrity, depicted in cartoons in the papers, on commemorative snuffboxes in the shops, and even in spoofs onstage.[10] He took no umbrage, but found a home and settled down in Paris.

After more than ten years of study and discussion, Gall was ready in 1808 to present his atlas of the brain, publishing the first in what would be a four-volume set on organology: *Anatomy and Physiology of the Nervous System in General and the Brain in Particular.** In it, he and Spurzheim identified twenty-seven organs within the brain. The first nineteen were found not only in humans but also in animals—an overlap that many traditionalists found distasteful. Even so, the descriptions used on Gall's charts were couched in terms of human propensities. The nineteen common faculties were:

1. Instinct of reproduction
2. Love of offspring
3. Affection, friendship
4. Instinct of self-defense, courage
5. Carnivorous instinct, tendency to murder
6. Guile, acuteness, cleverness
7. The feeling of property, the instinct to stock up on food, covetousness, tendency to steal
8. Pride, arrogance, love of authority
9. Vanity, ambition, love of glory
10. Circumspection, forethought
11. Memory of things and facts, educability, perfectibility
12. Sense of places, proportion
13. Memory and sense of others
14. Memory of words
15. Sense of language and speech
16. Sense of colors
17. Sense of sound, gift of music
18. Sense of connections between objects
19. Sense of mechanics of construction, talent for architecture

The organs that were found exclusively in human brains,

*The full title in French is *Anatomie et Physiologie du Systême Nerveux en Général, et du Cerveau en Particulier, avec des Observations sur la Possibilité de Reconnoitre Plusiers Disposi-tions Intellectuelles et Morales de l'Homme et des Animaux, par la Configuration de Leurs Têtes.*

according to Gall and Spurzheim, reflected traits that animals were not known to possess:

20. Comparative sagacity (wisdom)
21. Sense of metaphysics
22. Sense of satire, witticism
23. Poetic talent
24. Kindness, benevolence, gentleness, compassion, sensitivity, and moral sense
25. Faculty to imitate, mimic
26. Religion, knowing God
27. Firmness of purpose, constancy, perseverance, obstinacy[11]

Gall's list ascribed every impulse to the organs in the brain, leaving no aspect of behavior to anything as vague as spiritual guidance. Moreover, he suggested that with effort, the organs could be increased or reduced in size, and so in influence. Where physiognomy had concluded that humans had all of the "liberty of a bird in a cage,"[12] organology gave them the key to unlock that cage. There were limits, according to Gall. A person couldn't undergo a complete reversal, any more than that person could "exercise" a new skull into shape. However, by degrees, the organs would respond to a concerted effort; for example, piano study could enlarge the organ for musicality.

Napoleon didn't like it. He considered organology disruptive. In a letter to a friend, he wrote, "I contributed to ruin Gall. . . he and his like have a strong tendency toward materialism."[13] That was distinctly an unkind thing to say in the 1810s; it implied godlessness and irresponsibility, two traits that were often attached to Dr. Gall, unfairly. (The attack on religious grounds became so common that Gall devoted many of his later writings to affirmations that God was always part of the mind, however it operated physiologically.)

Once organology was launched in Paris, it became a staple topic in the city's famous salons, which radiated much of the influence in French society. However, Gall's theory was the basis of philosophical discussions, not medical ones. He ought to have been complimented. Philosophy, including the reason and rules for being, represented the pinnacle of France's own brainpower. But Dr. Gall was a man of medicine.

As the battle over organology continued to spark more anger than admiration, Gall may have been outmatched, good doctor though he was. When he tried to pull discussions of the mind into the world of medicine, he found himself on the defensive in a battle that was itself more consequential than any aspect of his theory. Medicine, with its understanding of physiology growing stronger, should have been ready to expand from the body to the being.

Though the controversy harmed Gall's reputation in some circles, his medical practice never suffered. Alert and informed, Dr. Gall was as popular in Paris as he had been in Vienna. In fact, many of the same aristocrats who jeered at him in public humbly sought his advice at the office. With science, gardens, and a great deal of money, Gall enjoyed his life in Paris and never wavered in his belief in organology. He died in 1828.

Organology is often cited as a starting point for modern brain theory, and even for psychoanalysis. However, it wouldn't be remembered as anything more than a topic of chatter in a chattering era, if Dr. Gall hadn't had a falling-out with his former assistant Johann Spurzheim in about 1812.

Gall had considered himself a scientist and nothing more, even claiming that he could support every aspect of his theory of organology with pure fact and observation. But Spurzheim believed that there was more to it than science. With an understanding of the composition of the brain, he was sure that people could help themselves or help each other to adjust in society. A moralist and humanitarian at heart, Spurzheim broke away from Gall, renamed the field "phrenology" to give it a new start, added a host of new organs to the original list of twenty-seven, and moved to England.

The English embraced Spurzheim's version of phrenology wholeheartedly, being less bothered than the French by philosophy and more open to reform than almost any nation on the continent. Practically anything that was popular in England was, in turn, a passion in America in the early nineteenth century, and phrenology was no exception, meeting with success from the moment of its arrival. Harriet Martineau, an Englishwoman who kept a journal of her tour of America in 1834, watched it happen. "The great mass of society became phrenologists in a day," she wrote.[14]

Edgar Allan Poe was a convert, and so were leaders throughout American society. The American medical community was heavily influenced by Gall's ideas.[15] Among the others who believed that there was something to it were Horace Mann, the educator, and Henry Ward Beecher, the minister. In both England and the U.S., phrenology attracted abolitionists, feminists, and those interested in the welfare of the lower classes. In those complicated times, when industrialization either trapped or frightened nearly everyone. phrenology was interpreted as offering a fresh sense of hope. Through it, one could understand and master the immediate universe, in personality, behavior, and even achievement. "Phrenology" became synonymous with a liberal outlook in America, as in Europe. It served as a precursor to the development of social science, not because of its own short-lived phenomenon but because of the many open-ended causes it helped precipitate.

Phrenology fell out of favor with physicians by the mid-nineteenth century, but it was not forgotten. Rather, its place was taken by other theories on brain structure and the localization of functions—ideas that marked a path leading to modern neurology. Even while medical historians debate whether organology was, in fact, the first step on that path, the best evidence of Franz Joseph Gall's role lies in the similarity of his ambitious goals and those of brain mapping efforts today. Two hundred years from now, perhaps those efforts will seem preposterous and awkward, but it is simply part of the long process of trying to understand how the brain becomes a mind.

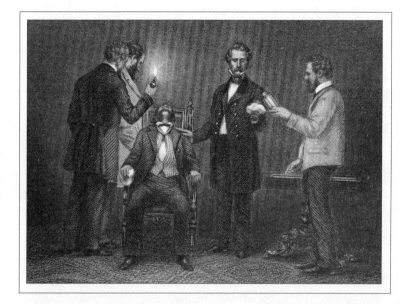

Horace Wells, William T. G. Morton, and Charles Jackson
ETHER FROLIC

S ulphuric ether evaporates easily at room temperature, giving off a thick, sickly sweet smell. It's a remarkable substance, despite the fact that for more than two centuries those fumes did very little for humanity beyond providing a fleeting moment of amusement for wealthy teenagers and a few debauched adults. Taken in the right dose and in a peppy frame of mind, ether made them giggle and dance; in smaller doses on top of a subdued mood, the fumes led to a more private nirvana. Nitrous oxide, which is a gas, had much the same effect. Neither did anyone any harm—but they didn't do them any good, either. It was all for kicks and laughs.

Ether might have stayed in the back parlor forever if it hadn't crisscrossed in history with nitrous oxide. Then, finally, it was brought by an unlikely escort into the operating room, where it was desperately needed during surgery. For thousands of years, patients and surgeons had waited without any real hope for that day to come. It was an era of horror and distress.

In 1833, a newspaper in Albany printed a rave review of a demonstration of nitrous oxide gas, presented by an itinerant lecturer named Dr. Coult of London, New York, and Calcutta.

As a matter of fact, "Dr. Coult" was not quite a doctor. He was Sam Colt, a tall nineteen-year-old from Connecticut who had already attended a boarding school in Amherst, dropped out of the merchant marine, quit his father's small textile factory—twice—

and, more important, completed designs for the first revolver-type pistol. He had indeed been to New York, London, and Calcutta (as a sailor), but he hadn't had to go nearly that far from home to learn about nitrous oxide: Whenever he and the chief chemist at the textile factory grew bored, they did what many laboratory workers of the day did—they indulged in a whiff of "laughing gas," as it was also known.

"The effect which the gas produces upon the system," reported the Albany *Microscope,* "is truly astonishing. The person who inhales it becomes completely insensible, and remains in that state for the space of about three minutes, when his senses become restored."[1]

Nitrous oxide was discovered and isolated in England in 1772. For years, it was regarded as a poison, but when Humphry Davy, at twenty-two, was put in charge of a research institution in Bristol and charged with finding medical uses for gases, he focused on nitrous oxide, writing a book on the subject in 1800. In it, he acknowledged that the first effect of inhalation was sublime—"an ideal existence," he called it. The second was laughter, and a desire to communicate some of the overwhelming joy unleashed by the gas. The third effect, after a large dose, was insensibility to feeling, which led Davy to suggest that it could probably be used to alleviate pain during surgical operations. [2]

Laughing gas did not belong to the world of medicine in the first part of the nineteenth century, however. The closest it came may have been the occasion when Dr. Coult was working the Mississippi and happened to be a passenger on a riverboat in the throes of a cholera panic. The passengers praised God . . . there was a doctor on their ship. They besieged Colt's cabin, and he had a panic of his own. Eventually, and very reluctantly, he saw the sick and doled out the only cure he knew, which was laughing gas. The patients all recovered nicely, leading them to spread word of a medical miracle and leading Sam Colt to conclude that none of them had had cholera in the first place.

Nitrous oxide was indeed a medical miracle, but after the first flurry of excitement over Davy's book, it was relegated to the world of chemistry as a mere listing among gases, and to the world of entertainment as the basis for a show. By that time, the medical world had been searching for relief from the pain of surgery for so long that it had given up real hope of finding such a thing. Like a patient worn down by constant distress—two thousand years of it—medical science had long since stopped looking for a cure-all. Pain was a part of life, and of surgery. One writer in the 1840s recalled a genial English bachelor he knew, an old friend of the family, who had had several deep disappointments over the years and borne them each gracefully, stoically. But when a doctor told him that he would have to undergo an operation, he went home, wrote out a will, and killed himself.[3] That wasn't a rare occurrence, or an unreasoned one in face of the horrifying prospect of surgery without anesthesia.

The fact that an anesthetic was so near at hand for a good half-century before it was finally utilized might seem a mystery. After all, Sir Humphry first suggested a surgical use for a gas that "was capable of destroying physical pain" as early as 1800.

Yet the men who finally promoted anesthetic gases were not "inventors"—they didn't even discover the painkilling and sleep-inducing qualities of the gases. Indeed, the achievement in the development of anesthesia was neither lofty nor scientific, it was only in bringing a fresh perspective to an old, unhappy problem. Noble as that is, anyone could have done it. But no one did until 1846: In the meantime, the specter of surgery was wrenching for doctors and patients alike. Genial old men killed themselves rather than face it. Before 1846, the greatest advance in surgery was generally considered to be the ligature, or stitch, introduced by a French military surgeon named Pare in the sixteenth century. Without it, even a successful operation was likely to result in the patient's bleeding to death or dying as a direct result of the methods used to close a wound, the most popular being cauterization by the application of hot irons. In the case of amputation, the stump might be dipped into boiling pitch to seal the blood vessels.

Exerting the newfound power to close a wound as well as open one, surgeons lifted themselves out of the ranks of mere barbers and into the more respectable realm of scientific medicine. Indeed, one of the surgical fads of the 18th century represents the luxury of what might be considered "optional surgery," and reflects the surgeon's sheer delight in his powers: trepanning (boring a hole in the skull) was intended to relieve pressures there. As a later physician remarked, "many a surgeon, in France particularly, thought as little of tapping a man's head as he would of tapping a wine cask."

Amputations continued to be the most common form of surgery, however, because while other physicians *practiced* medicine in the professional sense of the word, surgeons were limited to repetition of certain simple procedures to improve their knowledge and expertise. All operations consisted of a very few steps. Surgeons could develop ideas regarding complicated operations—and try them out on cadavers—but real patients could not withstand the torture of protracted cutting. Surgeons thus "practiced" in the sporting sense, improving their times, upon which reputations were based. One of the proud achievements of eighteenth- and early nineteenth-century medicine was the 54-second lithotomy (removal of stones from the bladder).

Sciences related to medicine—chemistry, biology, botany, zoology—advanced during the Age of Enlightenment of the late eighteenth century and led to new fields, including immunology, pharmacology, bacteriology, and nutrition. But surgical science could not move forward without the introduction of an effective anesthesic, a true painkiller.

Pain itself is a difficult entity to understand, existing as it does in the mind as well as at the source. A few early painkillers attempted to isolate the pain of surgery at the source by the use of tourniquets or even ice, to numb the area to be cut. Most, though, worked on the mind.

The avant-garde technique for painkilling in the early 1840s was called mesmerism, which was hypnotism in its earliest form. It had been developed in the 1770s by a wealthy Swiss, Franz Mesmer, who could induce a trance and control what he defined as the "animal magnetism" of patient by staring into their eyes and stroking their skin lightly, sometimes with a magnet, while he played the harmonica, incense wafting around the room. Mesmer was a showman—too much so for authorities in Vienna, who duly investigated his theories and then gave him twenty-four hours to vacate the city—but his basic method was reexamined in the 1830s, when a Scottish surgeon renamed it "hypnotism" and used it on patients facing surgery. Mesmerism could be amazingly effective in separating a person's mental state from the physical one, but it had its own peculiar drawback in that it was time-consuming, taking between forty-five minutes and twenty-four hours to produce a trance. It also had the drawback common to every single early painkiller: Its effectiveness varied widely from one person to another.

The same was true for narcotic plants used in surgery, from ancient times to the 1840s, including mandrake, hemlock, opium, and even lettuce. With the stronger of such substances, the unpredictability was double-edged and dangerous. The same dose that alleviated pain for some minority of patients did little or nothing for others. More typically, those facing surgery in the 1840s opted for the relative safety of alcohol—as much wine or whiskey as they could drink.

None of it was good enough. Accounts of operations performed before the advent of anesthesia are horrifying and Gothic in detail. At the hospital, operating rooms were located high up in towers or domes or in the cupola, so that other patients and people on the street couldn't hear what was going on. Once the patient was in place, usually strapped onto a table or in a chair, and perhaps given a last jigger of some liquor, the surgeon arrived, accompanied by five or six burly men. In one case recalled by an English surgeon, the patient wriggled out of the straps at the last minute and escaped, locking himself in the nearest bathroom. The surgeon himself broke down the door and dragged the terrified man back to the operating table. The New York *Tribune* described an amputation in detail in 1841: The patient was a young man, cradled tenderly the whole time by his father, and at the same time held roughly in place by the attendants. As the surgeons—there were two—made their cuts, the boy's screams were so full of misery that everyone who could left the room. The first part of the operation complete, the young man watched "with glazed agony" as the chief surgeon pushed a saw past the sliced muscles, still twitching, and listened as it cut through the bone with three heavy passes, back and forth. [4]

That need to look was oddly typical; a man who survived an amputation without anesthesia described it much later: "During the operation, in spite of the pain it occasioned, my senses were preternaturally acute, as I have been told they generally are in patients in such circumstances. I watched all that the surgeons did with a fascinated intensity. I still recall with unwelcome vividness the spreading out of the instruments; the twisting of the tourniquet; the first incision; the fingering of the sawed bone; the sponge pressed on the flap, the tying of the blood vessels, the stitching of the skin, and the bloody dismembered limb lying on the floor. These are not pleasant remembrances. For a long time, they haunted me. . ." [5]

The young New York patient's expression of "glazed agony" was also typical, though it boded even worse than wild screaming, because it reflected the wrenched mental state with which most patients emerged from the operating room. Sometimes it faded, but often it did not; many who recovered physically were permanently disturbed by the anguish. Those who gave reasons for opting against surgery often pointed to the probability that they would "never be the same again," a prospect that made life seem less worth fighting for. A military surgeon suggested that civil operations were even worse than battlefield injuries, which were at least borne in the passion of a cause, a form of self-hypnosis, he suggested. On the subject of severe pain, and the stunning spectacle of seeing and hearing—let alone feeling—one's flesh being cut apart, there were many people who justified the lack of an effective painkiller by asserting that such experiences were just as necessary to life as were joy and pleasure.

When Sam Colt set off on tour in 1832 with his bags of nitrous oxide, he joined legions of itinerant lecturers who served up worldly knowledge, an hour or so at a time, in every American town with a public hall. Or even those without them: Colt often set up his show on street corners. More entertaining than the average sermon, more educational than theatrical shows, the popular lecture—the documentary of its day—offered young people somewhere respectable to go at night.

After discussing the discovery of the compound, the lecturer would invite volunteers from the audience to come onstage for a snort. One handbill promised: "The effect of the Gas is to make those who inhale it either Laugh, Sing, Dance, Speak or Fight &c., &c., according to the leading trait of their character. They seem to retain consciousness enough not to say or do that which they would have occasion to regret."

Fashionable young people soon learned to skip the lecture, arranging instead for the lecturer, a doctor, or a pharmacist to bring a bag of nitrous oxide directly to parties held for the purpose. Some opted for a vial of sulphuric ether, the main attraction of an "ether frolic." The twentieth-century descendants of such middle-American hedonists would go in for bathtub gin or pot parties, with the difference that there was nothing illegal about an ether frolic. High spirits came on quickly and then wore off completely; the only real problem being that people sometimes suffered bruises or even broken bones during the mayhem of ether intoxication, without feeling it until later.

An Athens, Georgia, doctor named Crawford Long presided over many of the frolics around his hometown in about 1842, recalling of the first one that the guests "were so much pleased with the exhilarating effects of ether that they afterwards inhaled it frequently, and induced others to do so, and its inhalation became quite fashionable in this country, and in fact extended from this place through several counties in this part of Georgia."

It is part of the record on the development of anesthesia that Long successfully used ether as a painkiller on a handful of his patients during minor surgery in 1842–1843.[6] Though he never sought to publicize his technique, he has nonetheless been celebrated ever since, and even allowed a tinge of sympathy, for having achieved the great breakthrough, if only in isolation. Yet the doctor, kindly though he seems to have been, should be, in science, reviled: whether he was dithering or lazy, shortsighted or truly dim, his failure to project ether as anesthesia—outside of greater Athens, Georgia—only prolonged suffering worldwide for five years.

A better start was made December 10, 1844, but it was only a start.

Gardner Colton, a medical school dropout with a pleasant Vermont personality, was on tour, giving nitrous oxide lectures. When the tour stopped at Union Hall in Hartford, Connecticut, a dentist named Horace Wells happened to be among those who accepted the general invitation to try laughing gas onstage, where he seems to have belied the laughing gas promise that volunteers wouldn't do or say anything they would regret.

"He made a spectacle of himself," Mrs. Horace Wells reported.

One of the other volunteers, though, skinned his legs rather badly while cavorting under the influence of the gas. Sitting onstage, with his head just clearing, Dr. Wells asked the other volunteer if his legs hurt. The question itself was a surprise to the other man, because he didn't feel anything at all . . . yet the sight of his own bloodied legs was even more of a surprise. All at once, it occurred to Dr. Wells that the nitrous oxide gas could be used as a painkiller during dental work.[7] Dr. Wells claimed a few years later that his new thinking was based on analogies he found between the suspension of feeling during battle, and then again during drunkenness, and the need for such a state during surgery. Whether it was reasoning or idle observation that brought Wells to a moment of discovery in December 1844, it was that moment that led eventually to the adoption of anesthesia for surgery around the world. It was also the moment that, Wells's wife said in light of later events, brought her family "an unspeakable evil."

After the lecture, Dr. Wells asked Colton to bring a bag of nitrous oxide to the dental office, where a colleague would extract a wisdom tooth while Wells himself was under the influence of the gas. Colton obliged, and the tooth came out, not with the usual excruciation, but with a sensation that Dr. Wells described at the moment as "the prick of a pin."

Horace Wells was a high-strung man, a competent practitioner and well-meaning, perhaps to a fault. He had the right discovery, but he was not the right pioneer. After further experiments with nitrous oxide in dental surgery, he approached the nation's foremost surgeon, J. C. Warren of the Massachusetts General Hospital in Boston. Mass General, as it is commonly known, had opened in 1821, and was the nation's leading hospital for generations, pioneering ambitious medical specialties as well as areas now considered basic to good care, including continuing education, a strong nursing corps and the advocacy of cleanliness. Dr. Warren arranged for Horace Wells to demonstrate the painkilling qualities of nitrous oxide in a tooth extraction before a group of students. The procedure seemed to have been a success, until the very end, when the patient made a sound—some reports say that it was a mere groan, others that it was a full-blown cry. The patient later said that he felt no pain and didn't know why he'd made a sound. At the time, though, the audience interpreted the sound rudely and jeered the upstart dentist from the wilds of Hartford, Connecticut, calling his discovery "humbug."

Another pioneer might have jeered right back at the students, or at least put up a stronger defense than Wells did ("I took the bag away too soon," was all that he would say). Another pioneer would have persevered and made fuel out of derision. But Horace Wells literally slunk away from the operating room, and then retreated to Hartford, where he took to his bed and remained sick for most of the rest of the year.

The process of bringing anesthesia to surgery apparently required qualities that Horace Wells lacked. In Boston, on the way to his appointment in J. C. Warren's operating room, Wells had discussed his discovery with an old colleague, William Morton, who would prove himself exactly the right man to bring anesthetic gases to the front. He was everything that Wells was not: aggressive, savvy, selfish enough to be fearless, downright greedy, and lucky.

Only twenty-four, Morton already had an extensive résumé—or record. At nineteen, he had left his home near Worcester, Massachusetts, to try business in cities further west. In Rochester, Cincinnati, St. Louis, New Orleans, and finally Baltimore, he was a full-time con man and part-time wooer of rich women. Had he succeeded in either regard, he might not have returned to Massachusetts in 1843, tired and broke. With a small inheritance from an aunt, he turned to the study of dentistry, as one of a few students taken in by Horace Wells in Hartford. Forming a business partnership, he and Wells invented a kind of dental plate; before marketing it, they brought it to Boston to have it appraised by New England's leading chemist, Dr. Charles Jackson.

A year and a half later, when Morton set up an office in Boston, he was a married man who had promised his wife's parents that he would study to be a doctor. With that in mind, he undertook general medical studies, first under the tutelage of Dr. Jackson and subsequently as a part-time student at Harvard Medical School. When Wells arrived in Boston for his demonstration at Mass General in 1845, both Morton and Jackson met with him. That is when Wells divulged his ideas about using nitrous oxide in surgery. Neither Jackson or Morton evinced much interest, yet the idea obviously remained with them.

As a matter of fact, Morton later swore that Wells's stillborn discovery had nothing to do with his own search for a surgical painkiller. He maintained that he had heard the narcotic properties of sulfuric ether mentioned in one of his Harvard lectures, and thought out the possibilities of its use in surgery all on his own.

According to others, though, he was reminded of Wells's discovery in 1846 by an acquaintance from Hartford. Recognizing the commercial possibilities, in dentistry at the very least, he took action. First, he asked Dr. Jackson for a supply of nitrous oxide, in an elaborately offhand way. Jackson replied that he was all out of nitrous oxide, but that sulphuric ether would work just as well to calm nervous patients.

For his part, Jackson himself later insisted that he had developed sound theories on the use of ether gas in surgery all on *his* own—ideas, he said, subsequently lifted wholesale by William Morton. The actual story of the exchange of ideas among the three men, Wells, Morton, and Jackson, has been hopelessly tangled up ever since with the self-serving recollections each made in the grueling war they later waged for credit for the innovation.

According to the recorded events of 1846, though, William Morton did pursue a program of experimentation with ether in dental surgery that convinced him of the worth of ether in hospital, or "capital," surgery. As had Wells, he applied to John C. Warren for permission to demonstrate ether in an operation to be performed at the Massachusetts General Hospital. A hospital secretary wrote back, inviting him to "administer to a patient who is then to be operated upon, the preparation which you have invented to diminish the sensibility to pain."[8] The date set was October 16, 1846.

Morton was on the eve of triumph, and he knew it. Ether was going to be hailed as a monumental gift to humanity, and the man who controlled ether sales would be rich beyond reckoning—and he knew that, too. To make sure that he would be just that man, Morton added a few harmless impurities to ether, mostly in a vain attempt to disguise its sweet odor, and renamed the secret concoction Letheon. No one but Morton would know what was in Letheon. After all, a person couldn't patent plain ether gas. Letheon was another matter, one on which Morton took out a U.S. patent, in a loose arrangement with Jackson.

The Mass General operating "dome" was state-of-the-art for

1846, an immaculate table surrounded by cases of precision equipment. Admittedly, the sheer clinical competency of the place was compromised by two decorations staring out of one corner: an Egyptian mummy resting in its sarcophagus and a skeleton in a glass case. Yet their presence was not nearly as haunting to the proceedings as were the hooks and rings locked into the walls, left over from the past that would end that very day, when the strongest straps, and not wisps of gas, held patients in place.

Before a small audience of surgeons and students at Mass General, Morton was scheduled to administer Letheon to a man having a surface tumor removed from his neck. The moments leading up to the procedure were filled with drama—in part because Morton, true to form, arrived late. When he finally arrived, Dr. Warren stepped back from the patient, and said sarcastically, "Your patient, sir, is ready." Morton administered ether fumes through a tube as though he had been doing it all of his life, and not just a few weeks. After the patient had fallen into a deep sleep, Morton stepped back. "Your patient is ready, sir," he said to the haughty Dr. Warren. To the astonishment of all those present, the operation was completed in perfect silence—no groans, cries, or screams. Even Dr. Warren was humbled, which was as rare an occurrence as an epoch-making medical breakthrough. Addressing those in the room, Dr. Warren said in a hushed voice, "Gentlemen, this is no humbug."

The next day, Morton was just as successful, attending to a woman who was having a growth removed from her shoulder. After that, there was a delay of several weeks, as hospital administrators insisted on knowing the composition of Letheon. Morton cooperated and agreed that he would never charge Mass General for his concoction; on November 7, when he next appeared in the dome to give Letheon to a woman named Alice Mohan requiring the amputation of her leg, the galleries were jammed with doctors, students, and others who had heard of the new surgical phenomenon.

The whole atmosphere in the operating theater was charged with excitement and importance, so different than that which met

Wells in the same place three years before. And Morton was different, too, described by Daniel Slade, a doctor who watched the procedure, as "a man of commanding figure and appearance, very erect and dressed, as he usually was, in a stylish fashion peculiar to himself." A short time later, as the surgeons were tightening the ligatures that closed the wound on the woman's leg, she came to and had to be persuaded that the operation was over and that her leg was gone. With that, reported Dr. Slade, "the profound stillness and suspense which had hung over all present was broken by loud murmurs of surprise and admiration . . . Morton was the hero of the hour, and was regarded with feelings akin to those which might have been awakened had an angel suddenly appeared."[9]

Oliver Wendell Holmes Sr., the father of the Supreme Court Justice, was an eminent physician who rejoiced in the discovery of ether gas as a painkiller. In the aftermath of the Mohan operation, he sent a letter to William Morton, making a long-lasting contribution of his own: "Everybody wants to have a hand in the great discovery," he wrote on November 21, 1846. "All I will do is to give you a hint or two as to the names or name to be applied to the state produced and to the agent." From the Greek *an* for "in-" and *aesthesia* for "sensibility," Holmes created the words *anesthetic* and *anesthesia.*[10]

One afternoon in the middle of December 1846, a class of medical students in Glasgow were kept waiting for a scheduled anatomy lecture, and they were not patient about it, chanting and throwing things around the room. Finally, the professor appeared, grave with emotion, to tell them that the class was canceled. A ship had arrived that morning from Boston with news, "the greatest news that has ever been received by surgical science," he called it: A painless operation had been performed at the Massachusetts General Hospital. And an attempt would be made to repeat the technique that very afternoon at the Royal Infirmary in Glasgow. The students quietly followed their teacher to the Infirmary operating theater, which was already packed, to observe a successful operation under ether, albeit crudely applied through a sponge wrapped in a towel. The same sort of trial, surrounded by the same momentous anticipation, was repeated across Europe, and before the middle of 1847, ether was in use in hospitals around the world.

Chambers's Edinburgh Journal reported on a great many ether cases, including one in which a patient inhaled the ether gas for a few minutes, as he was directed to do, and then turned to those assembled to watch the operation, informing them that the process was "a piece of humbug" and a dismal failure. All the while, the surgeons were going about the operation on him, so complete was his insensibility to pain.

Europeans searched for sentiments lofty enough to convey their gratitude to America, the country that had given the world anesthesia. "A boon in favour of humanity," the *North British Review* called ether in May 1847. "Among the most eminent of benefits yet to be bestowed upon a suffering humanity," said *Chambers's Edinburgh Journal* in February of the same year. "A discovery which cannot but form an epoch in the world's history," the *Dublin Review* observed in 1850. And where humanity suffers the most—in wartime—anesthesia was credited in the course of the following twenty years with alleviating at least some of the misery left by battles in the Crimean and American Civil wars.

After the great discovery, however, onlookers were left with a problem: the discoverers. And the discoverers were left with an even bigger problem . . . each other. As soon as Charles Jackson saw William Morton being hailed as the "hero of the hour," he leaped forward with his own claim to have discovered the anesthetic qualities of ether. Horace Wells then piped up with his own claim to having originated the use of nitrous oxide as a painkiller and to instigating the thinking of Morton and Jackson along the same lines. Morton, fending off the other two, tried in vain to assert his patent on Letheon; when that effort collapsed—because everyone with a nose seemed to discern the presence of ether as the main ingredient—he began a new career, petitioning the U.S. Congress and pestering it for a stipend in lieu of lost profits from the unenforceable patent. The claims, counterclaims, sworn affidavits, and testimony on behalf of the three men filled thousands of pages in any arena that would entertain the debate, including the *Congressional Record,* the proceedings of the Academy of Sciences in France (special Ether Commission), the annals of American Medical and Dental associations, the official history of the Massachusetts General Hospital, and the popular press.

Those who had achieved a triumphant milestone in the well-being of humanity thus spent the rest of their lives debasing themselves with greed and jealousy.

It is odd to think that in delivering millions of people from suffering, they brought so much of it on themselves: All three died in a state of madness. Disappointed by the failure of nitrous oxide to rival ether as an anesthetic (though it would later become the standard treatment in dental surgery through the efforts of none other than Gardner Colton), Wells turned to chloroform, testing it on himself—not with the self-control of a scientist, but with the abandon of an addict. During a bender in New York in 1848, he was arrested for throwing acid on a prostitute. While in jail, he came to the sad and self-perpetuating realization that he was no longer sane. He wrote lucidly of his condition to his wife and then took his life by slitting a major artery in his leg, taking care to anesthetize himself first. [11]

Morton also died in disarray in New York City; diagnosed with nervous collapse after his last lobbying mission in Washington in 1868, he waited until the doctors left his home and then set off in a frenzy that ended when he jumped out of a moving buggy to plunge his head into a lake in Central Park. Dragged out of the water, he fell unconscious and died at the hospital the same day. [12]

Jackson went more quietly. Having divided his career between studious publications in geology and intense attacks on Morton's claim to having originated anesthesia, he was committed to an insane asylum near Boston, where he died in 1880, after seven years' confinement. [13]

Individually, Wells, Morton, and Jackson were ordinary men, but as a collision of ideas and emotions, they made a spark of brilliance for which a whole world had waited helplessly for a half-century.

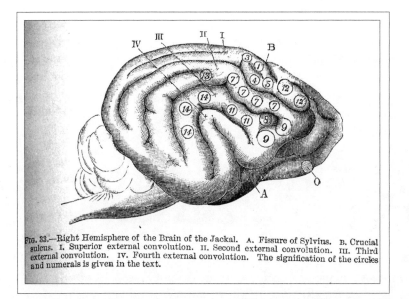

Fig. 33.—Right Hemisphere of the Brain of the Jackal. A. Fissure of Sylvius. B. Crucial sulcus. I. Superior external convolution. II. Second external convolution. III. Third external convolution. IV. Fourth external convolution. The signification of the circles and numerals is given in the text.

David Ferrier and
Frances Power Cobbe
HUMAN FEELING

T he Seventh International Medical Congress convened in London in August 1881 and drew three thousand doctors and researchers, a number that could not be overlooked as a sign that medicine was thriving in the Age of Science. Louis Pasteur was there and so was Rudolf Virchow, along with William Jenner, Thomas Huxley, Joseph Lister, William Osler, Robert Koch, and Jean Charcot.[1] Anyone who saw that medicine was surging and wanted to remain within sight of its future was in London for the meetings, which one writer has compared to a medical Olympics.[2]

The liveliest of the meetings was that of the Physiology Section, where the officers decided that the original format—the reading of papers—was a total waste of the opportunity offered by a gathering of good minds. Attendees could read the papers themselves anytime. The Physiology Section would hear a debate on the subject of "localization of function in the cortex cerebri." The cortex is the gray matter on the outer layer of the brain.

Friedrich Goltz of Strasbourg (which was then in Germany) was to start the discussion; he would be followed by David Ferrier of Britain. Ferrier, a Scotsman, had graduated from the University of Edinburgh, with further study in Heidelberg.[3] It was well known that the two held opposing views on the localization of brain function; however, their thinking was not based on mere speculation or intuition. Both were researchers of the first rank. The content of their theories—and the value of their science—

was a direct reflection of the best experiments they could conceive and perform successfully.

As Goltz explained, a new era in brain research had been launched in 1870 with the work of two German scientists, Gustav Fritsch and Eduard Hitzig, who exposed the brains of living dogs and stimulated different parts of the cortex with electricity, to see the effect.[4] With the current applied to certain areas, the dogs responded with a particular movement or facial expression. In other areas, there was no response. These results led Fritsch and Hitzig to conclude that the cortex was localized, or divided into parts, each with a different role. Goltz disagreed with that notion, explaining that the electricity might have affected tissue deeper inside the brain, under the cortex. In other words, Fritsch and Hitzig might have assumed that the charge had affected *outer* areas, when it really affected *inner* areas. To show that nothing had been proven with the electricity, Goltz also exposed the brains of living dogs, but he actually removed whole sections of the cortex. He then sewed the dogs back up to see how their behavior was affected by the ablation, as the removal of tissue is known. As his technique improved, he used a drill or a water jet to remove tissue; he reported that one dog survived after having eighty-six percent of its brain ablated. A thrill went through the audience when Goltz finished his talk by announcing that he had brought one of his ablated dogs to London and would not only open its head that very afternoon, so that the other delegates could see how much of the brain was gone, but kill the dog so that an autopsy could be performed during the Medical Congress.

Ferrier responded to Goltz with a description of his latest work, which involved monkeys. Using cauterization and antiseptic methods (as dictated by Lister), he and his colleague Gerald Yeo had learned to make very accurate ablations. Through their methods, they could effect any number of results, depending on what part of the cortex they removed.[5] Ferrier could paralyze certain limbs of a monkey, for example—and he matched Goltz's offer by offering to bring just such a monkey to the afternoon demonstrations.

That afternoon, Goltz displayed his dog, which could move around and make decisions despite the fact that part of its brain was gone. Showing off, Goltz put his fingers into the cavity left within its skull, and finished by promising to have the dog killed for the autopsy. Ferrier showed off two monkeys on which he had operated, one left partially paralyzed and one rendered deaf. He prided himself that he had the better experiments, saying of one that it reflected "a completeness never before reached." Therefore, in his estimation, he had the better science, which was ultimately the conclusion of those at the meeting as well. Ferrier also planned to kill his animals forthwith for the sake of the discussion.

The debate over localization was the high point of a lofty convention. Virchow and Charcot both chose to attend the Physiological Section session in favor of anything else going on at the Congress. The newspapers covered it as well. Ferrier and Goltz had given a rare glimpse into the work of the two most advanced neurological labs in the world.

The English public was left reeling by the privilege. People outside of the scientific world had seldom seen physicians strut so boldly the effects of vivisection, the term used to describe experimental surgery on living animals. The dog and monkeys that looked like interesting subjects to Ferrier, Goltz, and other researchers looked like defenseless victims of ghastly cruelty to many in the general public. An antivivisection group called the Physiological Society had been accorded time to make a presentation to the general meeting of the International Medical Congress,[6] but nothing that was said by the speakers lent as much urgency to the issue as the most calm and objective account of the Goltz-Ferrier debate.

The rather boastful comments that David Ferrier made about his work with animals would follow him during the rest of 1882, and even beyond that, as his work, which was at once both important and cruel, became a test for the attitude of English Victorian society toward medical science. Even while he was bringing out landmark texts such as *Functions of the Brain* and *The Localisation of Cerebral*

Disease, reformers in England were disseminating booklets with titles like *Professor Ferrier's Experiments on Monkey's Brains* and *Ferrieristic Brain Surgery: A Candid Condemnation.*[7]

The antivivisectionists, who would eventually try to put Ferrier in jail, were not only speaking out against the ghoulish abuse of animals—though that was the impetus that brought a remarkably powerful circle of people into the cause. The Archbishop of York, the Earl of Shaftesbury, Lord Chief Justice Coleridge, Robert Browning, Alfred Lord Tennyson, and Cardinal Manning were all involved in the campaign at the time when it focused on Ferrier. Underlying the antivivisection movement was a reaction to the expansive power of medical science in the late nineteenth century. Morally, medical research seemed to be positioning itself on its own plane. "Brutal carters and ignorant costermongers are brought to punishment for maltreating the animals under their charge," pointed out the Anglo-Irish writer and social philosopher Frances Power Cobbe, while "the mere allegation of a scientific purpose [puts medical researchers] above all legal or moral responsibility."[8]

The argument used to defend such research, of course, was that medical progress depended on animal experimentation. But actually that point, impressive as it was, sidestepped the issue of morality. As Stephen Coleridge, son of the Lord Chief Justice, put it, "Even if sanguine anticipation could be entertained that by torturing a monkey Mr. Bernard Shaw could be preserved to us for a hundred years, the issue would still remain whether it is right or wrong to torture a monkey."[9] The insistence on maintaining the principle that the end did not justify the means made the antivivisection uprising in Victorian Britain much more than an immediate defense of laboratory animals; it became a crucial part of the evolution of medical science. The antivivisectionists drew a line that said that not *everything* is all right in the name of medical science.

Altruistic intentions were not always present, anyway. "The idea of the good of Humanity was simply out of the question, and would have been laughed at," stated a scientist named George

Huggan of an animal vivisection lab in which he worked for a short time, "the great aim being to keep up with or get ahead of one's contemporaries in science, even at the price of an incalculable amount of torture needlessly and iniquitously inflicted on the poor animals."[10]

The sense of foreboding that underscored the antivivisection movement was that the temptation to experiment would not end with dogs and monkeys. Ambitious researchers, unchecked, would naturally turn to humans—but not, of course, their friends and neighbors. That would be a plot for a horror novel. In real life, the researcher would designate a group to dismiss, just as Victorian vivisectionists dismissed animals. That the temptation is real has been shown by Josef Mengele's experiments on Jews, Communists, Gypsies, and others in German concentration camps in the Nazi years; by the Tuskegee experiment that deceived African-Americans into participating in a study of syphilis from 1932 to 1972; and by the undisclosed testing of LSD on mental patients in New York City in the 1950s. In each case, the trick of prejudice had allowed the researchers to separate humans into two classes, and so dismiss the subjects of the research as being in an inferior category. Those are a few of the instances in which twentieth-century researchers performed human trials in the name of advancing science. The line of thinking that wipes all empathy from the mind of a researcher was the target of the early antivivisectionists. Without their introduction of a new morality to go with the new science, there would have been many more medical researchers using the ironic phrase "the good of humanity" as a license to perpetrate inhuman acts, on both animals and humans.

The antivivisection campaign started in the 1820s, and became an organized force in the 1860s. It arose in response to the work of two French physiologists, François Magendie and Claude Bernard. Magendie started work in about 1809. Though he was respected for making systematized observations of anatomy, his methods were abhorred, especially in England, since they put dogs through abject and unnecessary suffering. Sir Charles Bell, the most eminent anatomist of the day, detested Magendie's methods, speaking out against them and probably instigating the antivivisectionist movement. "I cannot perfectly convince myself that I am authorized in nature, or religion, to do these cruelties—for what?—for anything else than a little egotism or self-aggrandisement."[11] Even physicians in England who defended Magendie's experimentation on animals believed that he did go out of his way to inflict pain. Bernard, who began as Magendie's student, was the professor of experimental physiology at the Collège de France. A Massachusetts physician who studied there wrote that Bernard's dogs "were subjected to needless torture, for the mere purpose of illustrating well-known and accepted facts, capable of being taught satisfactorily by drawings, charts, and models . . . But when it is considered that these same experiments might have been conducted under the influence of an anesthetic, so as to minimize, if not remove, the needless suffering, this cold-blooded, heartless torture can only be characterized as contemptible and monstrous."[12]

Huggan, also a student under Bernard, described the dogs as they were brought up from the cellar where they were kept:

Instead of appearing pleased with the change from darkness to light, they seemed seized with horror as soon as they smelt the air of the place, divining, apparently, their approaching fate. They would make friendly advances to each of three or four persons present, and as far as eyes, ears, and tail could make a mute appeal for mercy eloquent, they tried it in vain. Even when roughly grasped and thrown on the torture-trough, a low complaining whine at such treatment would be all the protest made, and they would continue to lick the hand which bound them, till their mouths were fixed in the gag, and they could only flap their tails in the trough as a last means of exciting compassion.

"Were the feelings of experimental physiologists not blunted," Huggan concluded, "they could not long continue the practice of vivisection."[13]

Many Britons and Americans agreed and for that reason didn't trust the physiologists to govern their own activities. Gathering into groups in opposition, they tried to understand why medical researchers had the right to perpetrate agony on other living beings and to fathom where it would end. The English contingent was particularly well informed and influential. By 1875, even the respected journal *The Lancet,* a bastion of the medical establishment, favored some sort of legislation. With support from Queen Victoria and politicking by the Earl of Shaftesbury, English reformers finally succeeded in seeing a law passed limiting vivisection in at least some respects. Originally, they wanted cats and dogs exempted from all medical research, and pointed to Charles Darwin's assertion that dogs were endowed with consciousness to support their efforts to end the special cruelty visited on the animals through vivisection. Scientists including David Ferrier successfully resisted that clause.[14] In the law as it was passed in 1876, researchers had to be licensed for specific projects in animal research, they had to employ anesthetics in operations, and no animal was to be vivisected in order to demonstrate a fact already proven—to a group of students.

In general, medical researchers were bitter about the new law. Several, including Joseph Lister, moved to the Continent to pursue animal experiments without interference of any kind.[15] Gerald Yeo complained that "the delays in granting licenses and the general official procrastination, often amount to practical refusal and prohibition by loss of opportunities."[16]

The most ardent antivivisectionists were no more pleased with the new law. Frances Power Cobbe emerged as the leader of the dissatisfied wing of the movement, where all vivisection was regarded as unconscionable, licensed or not. Born in Ireland to the landed gentry—the upper-class segment nestled just below the nobility—she was a liberal reformer on some issues, including feminism, but a staunch conservative on vivisection, which she saw as a middle-class incursion into the ancient pattern of values that made England unique.

Cobbe was certainly a dog-lover, as practically any true Briton is, but she was not an outright defender of all animal rights. In that, she was unlike one of her contemporaries, who professed to having a "moral objection to exploiting the lower animals for our supposed service and for our use," an objection which forbade her from so much as riding a horse, milking a cow, or eating an egg—let alone eating the chicken it came from.[17] For her part, Cobbe had no objection to slaughtering farm animals for meat, because the death was quick and the habit of meat-eating consistent with the natural world. Her fundamental objection to vivisection lay with the subjection of an animal to cruel practices that were otherwise unknown in the natural world and therefore perverse in the modern one. She called vivisection "a *new vice*."[18]

Cobbe saw the rise of medical science as a middle-class phenomenon, and while that may smack of snobbery on her part, the rapaciousness she detected in late-nineteenth-century medical science was indeed more characteristic of openly competitive activities such as commerce and manufacturing than of science, as it had once been pursued.

"The *scientific* question of the utility of vivisection," wrote Cobbe, "has no more bearing on this moral and religious one than the richness of the spoil which we might rob from a foreign country determines the rightfulness of going to war to ravish it."[19]

Cobbe and her splinter group, the Victoria Street Society for the Protection of Animals from Vivisection, made a practice of perusing medical literature for reports of experiments and then comparing the projects listed with those officially licensed, according to the law. After the International Medical Congress in 1881, she happened to see that David Ferrier, the man of the hour, had not been issued a license to perform experiments on monkeys. Cobbe brought the infraction to the attention of the Home Office, which charged him with having "on the 4th of August and on divers other days, performed experiments, calculated to give pain to two monkeys, in violation of the restrictions imposed by the Vivisection Act."[20] It was a headline story, as Cobbe hoped. The British Medical Association immediately stepped in to pay Ferrier's legal costs.

Even before the trial began on November 18, a mob of students waited outside, howling and cheering; no one was quite sure which side in the dispute excited them, but the superintendent set up a police line to keep them on the street and out of the discussion inside. Cobbe and her associates were allowed in, however, and they watched the prosecution lay out the case against Ferrier. According to the attorney, Ferrier had not only failed to secure a license for his activities six months prior, but had kept several animals alive even after the anesthetic had worn off, for the sake of further experimentation on them.

The judge then remarked that if the acts were committed at least six months previously, he had no power to act, according to the law. The prosecuting attorney then turned to the debate at the International Medical Congress in August and contended that experiments had been conducted there as well. The defense responded with witnesses who testified that it had been Dr. Yeo, not Ferrier, who had performed the actual experiments on the monkeys. Yeo had a license that covered the type of work performed. While the prosecution tried to indicate that Ferrier personally directed the experiments, whether or not he picked up a scalpel, the judge replied that if he found Ferrier guilty for observing Yeo's actions, then he would have to find everyone in the audience at the debate guilty as well. Although the judge seemed to be sympathetic with the antivivisection viewpoint, he had no power to convict Ferrier. With that, the case was dismissed.

Both sides claimed victory. Cobbe had shown that her group was vigilant, even while proving that the Vivisection Law was not as strong as they felt it should have been. And Ferrier was free to do more experiments. Over the longer term, the factions within the medical establishment that had leapt to the defense of Ferrier solidified into an official organization to resist further inroads by the antivivisectionists.

Frances Cobbe continued to write philosophical pieces against vivisection and in favor of women's rights and her other causes. She died in 1904, having witnessed many fundamental changes to society since her girlhood in Ireland in the 1820s. She even succeeded in influencing a few of them. "In the death of Frances Power Cobbe," wrote her friend Frederic R. Marvin, "literature has lost an ornament and the world a true friend."[21] David Ferrier retired from research in the late 1880s, and worked as a clinician at a London hospital for the balance of his long career.[22] He died in 1928. His work in localization led directly to the first operation to remove a brain tumor in 1884.[23] By no means a villain in the history of medicine, he did come to symbolize one of its uneasiest dilemmas.

William Harvey was a flagrant vivisectionist, and so were many of the other medical pioneers included in this book. Without animal experimentation, perhaps it would have been more difficult or even impossible to develop the theory, of circulation, the kidney transplant, the heart-lung machine, germ theory and antibiotics. All of that makes the use of animals expedient, but does not necessarily make it right, which is why modern medicine is haunted by the sound of a wagging tail on a torture-trough—and an ethical problem that will not go away.

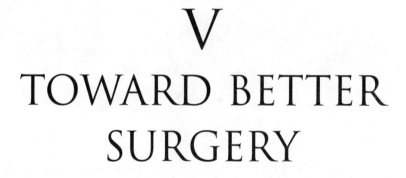

V
TOWARD BETTER
SURGERY

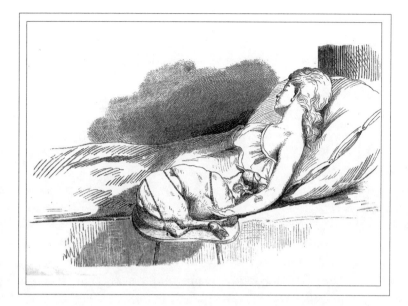

Jean-Baptiste Denis
TRANSFUSION OF MURDER

Three physicians hurried through the morning air of a town near Paris in February 1668, having just heard that a man named Antoine Mauroy had died during the night. Two of the doctors, Jean-Baptiste Denis and his assistant, Paul Emmerez, had attended Mauroy only the day before, and they were intent on performing an autopsy at the Mauroy household. While they might not normally have been in a rush at such a time, with the patient already dead, they knew that the Mauroy case wasn't over. It was far too public. Dr. Denis feared that the actual cause of death might never be known. He had heard rumors, though. And so he lost no time in getting to the house.

Madame Mauroy let the three men in, but when she heard why they had come, she made excuses and stalled for time. An energetic and forceful woman, she was the one who had convinced Denis to treat her husband in the first place, and she was in command on the day of his death. As soon as she could manage it, the doctors were herded out the door, without having examined the body or cut it open. By the time they returned with a judge's order, the widow had buried her husband. According to church law, it could not be exhumed.

With no hope of an autopsy, the Mauroy case became a blistering game of accusations, eventually embracing all of the active gossips in Paris—which meant most of the city in the 1660s. Mme. Mauroy called Dr. Denis a murderer; he in turn called her a murderer. The established doctors in France leapt to her defense, having motives of their own. The city's lawyers evened the match, tending to be more impressed with Denis than with a widow who seemed more relieved than bereaved.

Antoine Mauroy had been Denis's fourth experiment in blood transfusion. The doctor had pioneered transfusions on humans only the year before and still believed in his procedure. To him, it was crucial to prove that he hadn't killed Mauroy. Just what Denis had done to Mauroy grew into a cause célèbre, the biggest question of the year in Paris. The answer, which would come as much from the city as from the courts, would be a ruling on a tangle of grudge matches that had arisen over the case in French intellectual circles. Somewhere in the midst of them was Jean-Baptiste Denis's reputation. Even if Denis was innocent of a crime, he had to be stopped. He was a good physician, but too far ahead of his own knowledge on the subject of blood.

Jean-Baptiste Denis was a Parisian, probably born in the 1640s; the exact date isn't known. His father was a hydraulic engineer whose work can still be appreciated in the fountains at Versailles. Working directly for Louis XIV, the senior Monsieur Denis designed the pumping system that drew water from the Seine and delivered it to spray and gurgle in the palace fountains.[1] The birthdate of the son of such an eminent man would not normally be forgotten, but very few written records pertaining to Jean-Baptiste have ever turned up. As a young adult, he was generally regarded as a doctor, yet there is no evidence that he graduated from medical school. Later in life, when he was teaching math and philosophy, he attached the title of "professor" to his name, though again, there is no firm record that he earned a degree in either subject. Whether Denis did complete his studies or not, his lack of firm connections in French academic circles would eventually work against him. Nothing, however, could stop him from gravitating toward the newest ideas in the medical profession.

At least a decade before Denis was born, William Harvey had

given medicine a convincing description of the circulation of the blood. Harvey's breakthrough soon proved to be a foundation for more ideas, building on one another—small ones leading to great ones; great ones sometimes leading to nothing at all. Yet progress was ripe to occur more quickly than ever before. The same was true in the other sciences, for a variety of reasons. In the intellectual traffic jam of the mid-1600s, the sciences were being organized and inevitably, the exchange of ideas itself was becoming organized, too. To that end, British scientists formed a new kind of group in 1662, the Royal Society of London for Improving Natural Knowledge. To some extent, they were hoping to perpetuate the intellectual freedom of Oliver Cromwell's Commonwealth, which had ended in 1660 with the restoration of Charles II to the throne. London's political reversals may not have had much effect one way or the other on scientists in other countries, but the momentum that the times gave to scientific energy in Britain would soon reach throughout Europe.

The ascendency of the Royal Society was immediate and was the most obvious (and widely imitated) sign that British scientists were taking a new lead. The society's original intention was simply to provide a forum, a means to hear and be heard, through frequent meetings and the publication of a journal. The caliber of the discourse was high; the pioneering neurologist Thomas Willis was a member, and so were Samuel Pepys and John Locke. Isaac Newton joined only a little later and would serve as president.

With a combination of encouragement and competition stirring the Royal Society, the extension of the work of William Harvey was inevitable. Christopher Wren, the most prominent of the founding members, had already taken the first steps in that direction. Later in life, Wren would make his mark as the architect of St. Paul's Cathedral, but he joined the society as a professor of mathematics and astronomy. He was, more specifically, a math professor who had become fascinated with Harvey's theory and the wider implications of blood circulation. Wren had been inspired to try to turn the theory to practical use, injecting wine and beer into the vein of a dog in 1656 to see if it would get drunk.[2] It did. From that and further experiments, he concluded that the injection of medicine in humans was a practical possibility. Furthering Wren's experiment was a high priority within the newly formed Royal Society.

In the early 1660s, Richard Lower watched various medicines being injected into the veins of live animals and decided to make a trial with the ultimate medicine: blood. Lower was a Cornishman attending medical school at Oxford, and closely associated with Thomas Willis there. His experiment with transfusion took place at the end of February 1665. "I selected one dog of medium size," he wrote, "opened its jugular vein, and drew off blood, until it was quite clear from its howls and struggles that its strength was nearly gone.... Then, to make up for the great loss from this dog by the blood of the second, I introduced blood from the cervical artery of a fairly large mastiff, which had been fastened alongside the first dog."[3]

The first dog seemed to be in fine shape after the transfusion, leaving Lower only a few things left to do: sew up the dog's jugular vein, dispose of the body of the mastiff and announce his experiment to the Royal Society, which published an account in its journal in November and December 1666.

French scientists kept close track of developments across the Channel. In Paris, interest in new ideas was at least as high as in London, and even more hierarchical. A prosperous country well able to support layers of administration in almost every endeavor, France had long depended on the Medical Faculty of the University of Paris to judge innovations in healing. The faculty took a dim view of animal transfusion as it was practiced in England, not only because it was inhumane and rather ghoulish but also because it seemed unlikely to help humans. Though bloodletting was a cornerstone of medical treatment at the time, most physicians couldn't imagine taking the blood of one person and giving it to another. Medical lore offered an example of just such a procedure: Apparently in 1490, three little boys in Rome were given the promise of gold ducats in exchange for their good, young blood, which was to be administered to Innocent VIII, the old and ailing Pope. Whatever the exact procedure, all four participants died. The physician who masterminded the scheme had to flee for his life.

The story about Pope Innocent was widely known, something of a modern version of the Greek myth of Asclepius, who learned to use the blood of a Gorgon to bring dead people back to life. When Zeus found out that because of Asclepius, the underworld was running out of residents, he hit him with a thunderbolt. That put an end to the transfusions.

Perhaps the trepidation of the Medical Faculty members in Paris was a tacit admission of ignorance. Perhaps they sensed that there was a great deal still unknown about blood, knowledge that had to be gained before anyone could dare meddle with it; in that case, their position had a certain dignity. However, the faculty was also capable of taking a stand against experimentation with blood simply because the scientists gathered around Henri de Montmort were so excited by it. De Montmort, who held a high rank in the court of Louis XIV, had organized his own unofficial "academy" in direct contradiction to the old, conservative Medical Faculty. In 1666, he was able to secure royal patronage for his organization, which took the name it still carries today, the Académie des Sciences.

Jean-Baptiste Denis, an iconoclast who would not normally be anyone's disciple, fell in with de Montmort and became one of his protégés. In January, when Richard Lower's experiments with dogs were recounted in a French magazine, Denis read the article with rising excitement. Encouraged by de Montmort, he began his own research into blood transfusion.

Denis was determined to carry out a transfusion without harming either the donor or the recipient. His concern was partly expedient, since the gory destruction of the English dogs had gone a long way toward turning French opinion against the whole idea. But his eventual goal was to use transfusions on humans, and he certainly needed to do so with complete confidence of the well-being of both parties. The first trials took place in March 1667. Denis was able to trade the blood of three dogs around from one to another without harming any of them. Dogs share just one blood type, as do most other animals. (Humans, of course, have four different blood types, with further variations within each.)

Denis, and even more so the trio of dogs, was fortunate in having the services of Paul Emmerez, an expert surgeon who consulted closely on the procedure. Over the following months, the team not only repeated the dog-to-dog transfusions, but frequently demonstrated them in public, to the amazement of the many doctors who came to watch.

In all, Denis would perform over fifty animal transfusions, without damage to any of his subjects. He wrote copiously about his success, sometimes in journals, but also in privately issued pamphlets. A pamphlet in the seventeenth century was something akin to a website today; it was not edited, and so a person could use it to plead any cause without fear of interference. And like websites, pamphlets were widely read, readers being aware that while they were not necessarily as reliable as journals, they could be livelier. On the issue of blood transfusions, pamphlets carried the debate from each side to the people of the Paris.

To Denis, blood was a form of nourishment that could be exchanged between species.[4] Physiologically, he believed that transfusion was an extension of the instinct exhibited by many animals, including humans, to feed on the flesh of other species. As he came to that conclusion, he gave up on the idea of human-to-human transfusions in favor of taking the blood of animals for human patients, who, he hoped, would benefit from the finer qualities of the donor species: the energy of the dog, the gentleness of the sheep—and the absence of sin in all. A fundamental part of Denis's thinking was that many human conditions were caused by bad habits, vice, or outright sin and that animals, not being prone to any such unnatural inclinations, had purer blood that could only improve that of a troubled human.

When Dr. Denis heard about a patient who seemed to need a transfusion in the late spring of 1667, his first concern was what to prescribe—that is, which animal to tap. The case, in Denis's own account, came about suddenly that June:

> On the 15 of this Month, we happened upon a Youth aged between 15 and 16 years, who had for above two months been tormented with a contumacious and violent fever, which obliged his Physicians to bleed him 20 *times,* in order to assuage the excessive heat.
>
> Before this disease, he was not observed to be of a lumpish dull spirit, his memory was happy enough and he seem'd cheerful and nimble enough in body; but since the violence of this fever, his wit seem'd wholly sunk, his memory perfectly lost, and his body so heavy and drowsie that he was not fit for anything. I beheld him fall asleep as he sat at dinner, as he was eating his breakfast and in all occurrences where men seem most unlikely to sleep.[5]

As Denis put it, the boy passed his days in "an incredible stupidity." He astutely recognized that well-meaning doctors had simply taken too much blood; they had treated the fever by giving the boy acute anemia. Denis's basic inclination was to replace some of the lost blood, a possible use for transfusion that had never occurred to his rivals in England. To treat the "lumpish" boy, Denis took blood from him in the amount of three to five ounces. "At the same time," he wrote, "we brought a *Lamb,* whose *Carotis Artery* we had prepar'd, out of which we emitted into the young man's Vein, about three times as much of its Arterial blood as he had emitted into the Dish."

"We caused him to lie down on his Bed," Denis continued, "expecting the event; and as I asked him now and then, how he found himself, he told me that during the operation, he had felt a very great heat along his arm." That evening, the boy was up and around, on his way to a complete recovery—"and he hath no longer that slowness of spirit or heaviness of body," Denis said. The event he had "expected," the calamity hovering over any initial experiment, had failed to materialize.

Denis's next trial did not arise from a medical emergency. For the sake of science, he recruited a forty-five-year-old man, a perfectly healthy sedan-chair carrier, who agreed to undergo the transfusion for a small payment. A young sheep was used as the blood donor, in part to see if the man's coarse personality would become more lamblike as a result. The transfusion was a success to the extent that the man suffered no ill effects. However, his personality didn't exactly change. In fact, he jumped up when the transfusion was through and slit the lamb's throat. He wanted the fleece.

The family of a young Swedish count who had fallen gravely ill during a visit to Paris desperately solicited Denis's help, imploring him to perform a transfusion as soon as possible. The patient briefly improved, but within hours, he was dead; the cause was intestinal disease, according to an autopsy. The incident had little effect on developments surrounding transfusions.

Overall, the year 1667 belonged to Denis. His success with transfusions had garnered the attention that he undoubtedly craved, although it pitted him against the powers of medical practice in Paris in all their many guises. The Medical Faculty, of course, was especially leery. Cranking our pamphlets and articles, Denis was too busy to perform many more transfusions during 1667. In London, meanwhile, Richard Lower hired a recent Cambridge graduate named Arthur Coga to be the subject of his first animal-to-human transfusion in November 1667.[6] At the time, Lower was sure he was the first person anywhere to attempt a transfusion involving a human. The initial animal-to-animal experiments had revolved around the Royal Society, after all, and he had no reason to believe that so much progress had been made in France. Neither did anyone else, and so the Coga procedure was a public event, well attended in London.

Coga was a strange fellow, "a little cracked in the head,"[7] according to one account, and his elders felt that a transfusion couldn't possibly do his personality any harm, though they were curious to see how it would affect his body. The blood of a sheep flowed into Coga's veins, just as planned, and when it was through, Coga walked away, with twenty of the easiest shillings he'd ever earned. The Royal Society was quite openly pleased with the way it had shown the way in human transfusions, until the members learned a few weeks later that Jean-Baptiste Denis had already been performing transfusions on humans for six months.

The problem with the animal-to-human transfusions of 1667 was not that they failed disastrously. Quite the opposite. The problem was that they worked. They shouldn't have; animal blood is incompatible with human physiology. If the seventeenth century doctors had known anything about the composition of blood, they might have known that, but actually they knew nothing more about it than old Asclepius had—and he was charbroiled for dabbling in what he didn't really understand. By all that is known today, the animal blood should have been rejected by the handful of subjects who had it flowing in their veins. Some modern physicians suggest that the amount of blood transferred was actually less than originally thought, though the reporting on the various experiments seems to be accurate on other counts. Another suggestion is that the cells in the transfused blood were destroyed before they could present a problem to the recipient.[8] In any case, the transfusions were a kind of bubble in the medical world—buoyed by talk and filled with hope. But no one really understood them.

As of December 1667, Madame Mauroy, described as a "young gentlewoman," had been married for about a year to a house-servant named Antoine Mauroy. Some years before, when Mauroy was about twenty-six, he had suffered a broken heart that nearly killed him, bringing on a "phrensy." Some people have conjectured that it was no romantic tragedy that caused Mauroy's frenzies, but syphilis. Still other theories circulated at the time. At any event, by the age of thirty-three Mauroy was recovered enough to move on and get married. By turns, however, his fits of madness returned, and his new wife later said that when he was out of his right mind, he beat her. A string of employers also claimed to have lived in fear of Mauroy when he was on a tear. As a consequence, Mme. Mauroy took it upon herself to contact Dr. Denis and ask him to attempt a blood transfusion. Denis consented. On December 19, the deranged young husband received his first dose of calf's blood, and a few days later he received another.[9] The result was encouraging, as the man was returned to a lucid and quite likable state, though on the second occasion, he did exhibit signs of minor blood poisoning, such as blood in the urine.

Naturally, Denis wrote a pamphlet all about the case, and went to press with it in February. But even as the ink was drying on the pages boasting of success, Antoine Mauroy was on another rampage. His wife responded by following Dr. Denis everywhere, from town to town on calls around Paris, begging him to try another transfusion. She even bought a calf and had it standing by at her home.

Dr. Denis no longer wanted to attend the Mauroys, though. He had heard rumors that Mme. Mauroy was slowly poisoning her husband by putting powders in his food. Some people suggested that the poison was causing the madness. However, she was nothing if not convincing, in addition to being quite obviously desperate, so Denis reluctantly summoned Dr. Emmerez. The two of them went through the motions of administering a third transfusion, but by then Mauroy was no longer cooperative and no transfusion took place. Denis and Emmerez, feeling that they had done everything they could, returned to their inn. It was the next morning that they heard that Mauroy was dead.

Denis immediately planned an autopsy to examine the dead man's digestive system, in order to look for signs of poisoning, but it was too late. As quickly as Denis, Emmerez, and a third physician rushed to the Mauroy home, news was spreading even more nimbly to Paris and beyond. The word was that Jean-Baptiste Denis had killed a patient, that transfusion carried death into the veins.

Denis fought back, charging that the widow had been poisoning Mauroy all along and had only enticed him into giving transfusions as a cover for her own murderous plot. The Faculty of the Medical School at the University of Paris immediately charged to Mme. Mauroy's defense. According to observers, they may even have coaxed her into leveling charges of manslaughter on Denis, but that insinuation may have been slanderous.

In fact, it was all slander. A few months later, a court decided in Denis' favor, exonerating him of any role in Mauroy's death. Justice never focused as clearly on Mme. Mauroy. A preliminary investigation showing that she had indeed put powders in his food was supported by further proof that she had purchased cyanide in Paris. If she arranged the transfusions simply to cover up a murder, she might have done a great disservice to medicine. Or she might have helped it immensely.

By official edict, France, Britain, and the Roman Catholic Church all effectively banned the transfusion of blood in the wake of the Mauroy case. It would be more than 150 years before transfusions would find favor in medicine again.[10] That was not to be regretted, though. Over the coarse of those 150 years, the microscope was continually improved and gases such as oxygen and carbon dioxide were recognized, giving physicians a basis for understanding the composition of blood. It wasn't until that knowledge led to the identification of blood types and an understanding of what blood is and what it does that the practice of transfusion could be developed.

After the Mauroy murder trial, Jean–Baptiste Denis practiced medicine in Britain for a short time, even serving in the court of Charles II. However, when he returned to France in 1673, he gave up his medical practice for good. With his experiments in blood transfusion, he had undoubtedly seen the future. That didn't mean he could be a part of it.

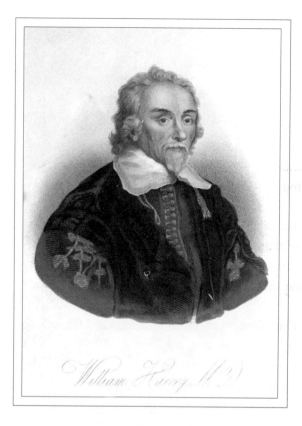

William Harvey
MASTER OF THE SYSTEM

I n 2000, an otherwise healthy young Welsh woman collapsed in London's Heathrow Airport, having just arrived on a flight from Australia. She died almost immediately.[1] The cause of death baffled her companions, but held no mysteries for officials at the hospital nearest to Heathrow Airport. They knew it as deep vein thrombosis, a condition that swept into the jargon as "economy class syndrome."

When people sit still for long periods, as on an airplane, the circulation of the blood is likely to slow down. Pools may even collect in the larger veins of the legs, with clots forming in the stagnated blood: That is deep vein thrombosis (DVT). DVT is not all that rare—a study based in London found that more than 3 percent of the people in a test group developed DVT during the course of an eight-hour flight to New York.[2] And in and of itself, DVT isn't particularly harmful, either. If the clot disintegrates as gradually as it formed in the first place, then it will cause nothing more disastrous than a dull ache in the leg. However, in rare cases, the clot breaks loose intact—and that can have serious consequences. Joining the flow of the bloodstream, it will travel to the upper part of the body where, if it doesn't dissolve en route, it can cause a blockage in the lungs. That blockage, known as a pulmonary embolism, is tantamount to being strangled from the inside, and can be lethal.

Statistically, the number of people who suffer a pulmonary

embolism as a result of air travel is infinitesimal. According to records at Charles de Gaulle Airport in Paris, only fifty-six passengers out of the 135.3 million who used the airport from 1993 to 2000 developed the condition, and not all of them died.[3] The actual numbers may be small, but the sense of tragedy is towering, as death seems in every case too high a price for the innocent mistake of sitting still too long. In the wake of the death of the young woman at Heathrow, travelers began to look out for themselves. The goal was simply to move around enough to keep their blood circulating, not necessarily an easy task at 35,000 feet.

Until 1628, the blood did not circulate—or at least it was not presumed to do so. Instead, it was thought to push forth from the liver, as needed. The news that it rode through the veins and arteries on a circuit was delivered that year in a book written by William Harvey of London. The book, *De Motu Cordis,* may have been a brilliant contribution to medical literature, but it was a mediocre piece of publishing—too hastily produced even to allow Harvey to correct typos and other small errors. It was akin to a cheap paperback, but that didn't stop people both within the medical world and outside of it from reading *De Motu Cordis,*—which is Latin for "the motion of the heart." They were fascinated not only by the subject matter, but by Harvey's silken sense of self-confidence.

In the book, Harvey explained the role of the heart in pumping blood in a grand loop through the vital organs, then on to other tissue and back again. It was an illumination that medicine's more radical theorists had been flirting with for the better part of a century. In their wake, the medical world as a whole had been tempted toward it several times, only to shy away each time to remain snug in the shadows of ancient learning.

With William Harvey, though, there would be no turning back. Beyond pushing the medical world to a new level of comprehension regarding the specific process of circulation—which he certainly did—Harvey introduced a whole new sense of system into physiology.

Even though Dr. Harvey brought a commandingly fresh outlook, no scientist, however dispassionate, arrives on the scene of research without some frame of reference, some imprint on the mind to give a sense of order to the chaos of all those things not known. While a great scientist changes the perception of what is actually known, the sublime ones go even further and change the perception of what isn't known, shifting the predisposition of the scientific mind to reach for a fresh wave of discoveries.

In Harvey's time, that generalized scientific mind was benefiting from just a such a shift. The impetus originated in the field of astronomy, in which the concept of the solar system, first suggested by Nicolaus Copernicus in the mid-1500s, was being championed by Galileo Galilei. As a teacher and writer in the early 1600s, Galileo met with official damnation for espousing Copernicus's idea that the earth was not the center of the universe; he would ultimately be jailed for his scientific convictions. In Germany, Johannes Kepler was also developing the Copernican theory, producing a set of laws that not only affirmed the structure of the solar system, but described the orbit of the planets. Late in the same century, Isaac Newton proved Kepler's laws on a mathematical basis.

While this transformation in astronomy was of immediate interest to astronomers and physicists (and of practical use to mariners), the fundamental thinking behind it gave scientists in all fields a new template—a new way to approach a realm of ignorance that lay just out of reach. An investigation of a problem didn't have to start with the individual components. If it did, then the earth would naturally be assigned the position of greatest importance in the heavens, at least to any self-respecting earthling who was formulating a theory. Instead, Copernicus, Galileo, Kepler, Newton, and others of that exciting era projected the idea that it was not the elements within a problem but the *relationship* between those elements that described a system—a system reflecting the broadest possible understanding.

That shift in outlook formed the backdrop of William Harvey's career. More than any other figure, he was the one who brought the new scientific outlook into medicine, then the most tradition-bound of all the natural fields. That accomplishment alone turned Harvey into a veritable demigod in his own field. "William Harvey resembles Napoleon," observed A. Dickson Wright in 1961, "in that his life is constantly being written and new material incorporated in each fresh effort to recall his greatness."[4]

Harvey was from Folkestone, on the southeastern coast of England at the narrowest part of the English Channel. He was apparently born on April 1, 1578, although well-meaning biographers later switched the date to April 2 to save him from being an April Fool.[5] His father, Thomas, was a merchant whose family could be traced to Walter Hervey, a mayor of London in the thirteenth century, commonly known as "the Pepperer" because he had started out as a grocer. Less is known about William's mother, except that she was a notably kind-hearted woman named Joan Halke Harvey.[6] Thomas Harvey was successful in business and provided well for his nine children—two daughters and "a week of sons," as one biographer put it. All of the other younger boys were drawn to commerce, like their father (and like him, they would prosper), but William, the eldest of the sons, was consumed by learning, and at fifteen, he was sent to Cambridge University. After briefly considering a career in the church, he chose to study to be a doctor and upon graduation, he enrolled in a medical course at Padua, the leading university town of Italy. At both schools, William Harvey was a conspicuous success, popular with his classmates and regarded as a brilliant student by his teachers.

Physically, Harvey was small and trim, with jet-black hair and small, nervous eyes. Though he maintained a steady personality in most situations, he had a coiled energy within and a hair-trigger temper. His first biographer, John Aubrey, made note of the fact that Harvey wore a dagger at his belt, long past the time when it was fashionable for gentlemen, and he fingered the handle during conversation as if he were always at the ready to use it. Although

Harvey certainly didn't suffer fools gladly, he did suffer his colleagues with remarkable aplomb, was known for his loyalty and counted a wide number of friends throughout his long life.

A student like Harvey, intent on physiology, couldn't have done better than to pursue his interests at Padua in 1597. Vesalius had studied there, sixty years before, and when Harvey arrived on campus, Hieronymus Fabricius de Aquapendente, one of the leading anatomists in Europe, was a professor. At sixty, Fabricius was a wise mentor, but one caught at the ankle, as it were, by the very traps Harvey would manage to sidestep. In frequent demonstrations at Padua's sumptuous operating theater, Fabricius taught his students to note the valves in the blood vessels—his special area of expertise. They should have indicated to him the movement of the blood. However, Fabricius stopped short of any conclusion so controversial.

Like most physiologists of the time, Fabricius did not think it wise to counter the established authority, which rested largely with two men, Aristotle and Galen. It might be said that Aristotle (384–322 B.C.) was at the very epicenter of the glory of Greece, as the student of Plato and, later, the teacher of Alexander the Great. He embraced a wide array of fields, including biology, and even founded a few, including logic. Although he pointed out in one of his books that "blood beats or palpitates in the veins of all animals alike all over their bodies,"[7] he couldn't discern any movement by that beating, and couldn't make very much sense of the heart, to which he attributed three chambers rather than two. In truth, the heart is something like a jellyfish in that it is a tricky business to assign it any definite properties, especially when it is inactive (as in a cadaver).

Claudius Galen (c. 130–c. 200) was the eminent physician of Rome in his time, attending, among others, Emperor Marcus Aurelius. He was also a prolific writer, producing five hundred essays on medicine, eighty-three of which survived into the Middle Ages. Galen was not reluctant to vivisect (cut open living animals), a pursuit regarded as intolerably cruel by most of his predecessors. He allayed any guilt he might have felt by describing how he would bind the wound afterward and, in at least some cases, watch as the animal went on living.

However impressive Galen's descriptions of the beating heart were to generations of followers, and however accurate his understanding of the role of blood in carrying fresh air into the body and exhausted "soot" out, his speculation on the major organs was flawed. He considered that food was digested in the stomach and then passed for further refinement to the liver, where it emerged in the form of blood. The lungs served the liver by adding air to the blood. The heart was a kind of overflow valve. That is a vastly simplified version of Galenic anatomy, which was, by and large, a mixture of about 85 percent superb observation, 15 percent pithy inference and 5 percent flight of fancy, very officiously expressed in order to rationalize the occasional gaps between that which he observed and that which he inferred. Some medical treatises, even to this day, are composed of the same three ingredients, and sometimes in about the same proportion. In other words, Galen was much more right than wrong, and that is all that can be asked, in retrospect, of anyone willing to take on the boldest researches of scientific inquiry. It wasn't his fault that the treatises he wrote in the second century stood as the centerpiece of a sadly static medical world more than a thousand years later.

Galen and a few later physiologists were aware, to some extent, that the blood moved. Several of them were considered modern thinkers in 1600, when Harvey was at school in Padua. Vesalius was one; Fabricius should have been another. If teachers such as Fabricius shrank away from formulating a theory that seemed well within reach, it may have been that they just didn't know how close the truth was.

In the book *Circulation and Respiration* (1964), Mark Graubard gave a sense of perspective to the dilemma that preceded William Harvey: "Like Galen," Graubard wrote, "Vesalius vaguely presupposes some kind of blood flow, but the scheme is as unformed in his mind as are our contemporary ideas on the nature of memory, the meaning of sensation, the meaning of attraction, the nature of a field of force, the causes of the rise and fall of nations, and the making of a criminal. Future scholars may wonder how we failed to see what seems so clear to them. Yet we continue to rely on our beliefs, unaware of possible inconsistencies. Galen and Vesalius were in the same position. They knew that the blood was in a state of flow, and they knew that it followed specific courses in and out of the heart, but they were unable to conceive of the circulatory mechanism as a whole, as we do, partly because they were satisfied with their own assumptions and explanations."[8]

Satisfaction, intimidation, or a profound lack of preparation—none of the things that held back other admittedly brilliant scientists would count at all in the makeup of William Harvey.

As a student in Padua, accustomed to watching dissections of human cadavers, Harvey would sometimes walk through the market streets of town on his own time, and he couldn't help noticing the live fish in the mongers' stalls, still flopping around gasping for breath. He began to buy freshly caught fish, rushing them back to his rooms, where he performed vivisections in order to observe the workings of living hearts. Before long, he took to going on nature walks, mostly to catch an even wider array of specimens.[9] At the same time, Harvey was attending lectures by Galileo, who was then attached to the University of Padua and he was well aware of the revolution unleashed in the science of astronomy.

Harvey's firsthand observations of live animals, laid over an awareness of partially correct theories on blood circulation that were known but discarded at Padua—and sparked by Fabricius's obsessive interest in the function of valves—led at some point to his realization that blood flows in a circuit through the body. The exact moment of the inspiration has never been fixed.

A colleague once asked Harvey to recollect the process by which he came to understand that blood circulated. He could recall the process, but not the date. "He answered me," wrote the friend, Robert Boyle, "that when he took notice that the Valves in the Veins of so many several Parts of the Body were so Plac'd that they gave free passage to the Blood Towards the Heart, but oppos'd the passage of the Venal Blood the Contrary way: He was invited to imagine, that so Provident a Cause as Nature had not so Plac'd so many Valves without Design; and no Design seem'd more probable, then that, since the Blood could not well, because of the interposing Valves, be sent by the Veins to the Limbs; it should be Sent through the Arteries, and Return through the Veins, whose Valves did not oppose its course that way."[10]

The theory probably solidified in Harvey's thinking after he returned home to begin practicing medicine in London, performing his own experiments on the side,[11] but whatever the time frame, he didn't immediately publish any sort of book to trumpet his breakthrough. William Harvey was wise in the ways of human politics—being the son of a merchant may have helped in that respect—and it would take even longer for him to prepare for the announcement than it had to produce the discovery in the first place. Still, waiting was dangerous. Someone else might beat him to the idea, at least in the public view, but that was not much of a concern in Harvey's day, and certainly not in Harvey's mind. On the contrary, putting one's name on any departure from the medical canon in the seventeenth century was fraught with risk. For the time being, he settled down, married well (the daughter of Queen Elizabeth's personal physician), and impressed practically everyone he met with his sharp intellect, even while quietly confiding his theory of blood circulation to a few close friends. Even in choosing London as his home, Harvey was fortunate, since London was the fastest-growing city in Europe. It was also one of the most disease-ridden, which put special pressure on its doctors and encouraged a receptive attitude toward new ideas.[12] Almost as soon as Harvey began to build his fashionable practice, he became an active member of the reigning professional group in his field, the College of Physicians of London.

In 1616, at the youthful age of thirty-seven, Harvey accepted an invitation from the College of Physicians to deliver the Lumleian Lectures (named for a benefactor named Lord Lumley). It was one of many honors accorded the eminent, and eminently presentable, William Harvey, and it was the one that would ultimately prove the most important. The Lumleian Lectures on the subject of surgery were intended as a form of continuing education for practicing physicians; focusing on a different topic each year for six years, they included annual dissections that were usually very well attended.

Ever since college, Harvey had continued his research into the circulation of the blood, gaining a lasting reputation as a rather brutal vivisectionist. He cut into living animals of all kinds in order to see how they functioned and what kept them alive. Unlike Galen, he didn't seem to care one whit about the horrors he inflicted, or try to sew up and revive the animals he had thrust into a screeching hell. It was in the name of science, and the best that can be said is that the animal experimentation was not undertaken in vain: Harvey was an extraordinary researcher and recorded his observations in minute detail. Ironically, he liked animals and fancied that there was practically nothing he didn't know about their anatomy. That conceit was the basis of a story he once told:

A parrot, a handsome bird and a famous talker, had long been a pet of my wife's. It was so tame that it wandered freely through the house, called for its mistress when she was abroad, greeted her cheerfully when it found her, answered her call, flew to her, and aiding himself with beak and claws, climbed up her dress to her shoulder, whence it walked down her arm and often settled upon her hand. When ordered to sing or talk, it did as it was bidden even at night and in the dark. Playful and impudent, it would often seat itself in my wife's lap to have its head scratched and its back stroked, whilst a gentle movement of its wings and a soft murmur witnessed to the pleasure of its soul. I believed all this to proceed from its usual familiarity and love of being noticed, for I always looked upon the creature as a male, on account of its skill in talking and singing . . . until . . . not long after the caressings mentioned, the parrot, which had lived for so many years in health, fell sick, and by and by being seized with repeated attacks of convulsions, died, to our great sorrow, in its mistress' lap, where it so often loved to lie. On making a post-mortem examination to discover the cause of death I found an almost complete egg in its oviduct . . .[13]

There were surprises in any investigation. However, Harvey had devoted enough time to the study of circulation to introduce it as a verified fact in his Lumleian Lectures. Even there, among respectful colleagues, he did not rely on his own word. His hand-written (or, in the case of his appalling penmanship, hand-scratched) lecture notes carry the reminder, "Not to prayse or disprayse [other anatomists]; all did well."[14] He was also determined to let the anatomy itself carry his point, and so he made notes to himself to emphasize thorough observation and to make sure that everyone could see what he was doing during the Lumleian dissections. He also reminded himself to "speak playnley," and made his lectures lively with references to exotic birds in the Royal Collection in St. James' Park, London street names, football, bear-baiting, ballet, tumblers, rope-makers and a certain man who could pop the buttons off his shirt simply by inhaling deeply.[15]

As to the function of the heart, Harvey identified it clearly as a pump, telling his listeners that blood moved through the aorta "as by two clacks of a water bellows to rayse water."[16]

Dr. Harvey's reputation as an intellect, but an attractively lively one, brought him to the attention of Charles I, who was crowned king of England in 1625. While the doctor was often asked to tend to the ailments of the king and royal family, he also entered into Charles's inner circle, as a personal friend.

In 1628, Harvey was ready to publish his astounding theory of blood circulation. From the first, he was braced for criticism. "I did open many times before," he wrote to the College of Physicians, "my opinion concerning the motion and use of the heart and Circulation of the blood new in my lectures; but being confirm'd by ocular demonstration for nine years and more in your sight, evidenced by reasons and arguments, freed from the objections of the most learned and skillful Anatomists, desired by some, and most earnestly required by others, we have at last set it out to open view in this little Book . . ."[17]

Harvey was perfectly aware that the publication was a dangerous venture for anyone, but especially for someone with plenty to lose in terms of stature and appointments. In the preface, he acknowledged that, to the extent that he had already spoken about the circulation of the blood, "these views, as usual, pleased some more, others less: some chid and calumniated me and laid it to me a crime that I had dared to depart from the precepts and opinions of all anatomists . . ."[18]

Harvey's grand departure was the book called *Exercitatio anatomica de Motu cordis et sanguinis in animalibus* (which translated as "An Anatomical Dissertation on the Motion of the Heart and Blood in Animals"). Commonly called *De Motu Cordis,* it was only seventy-two pages in length, divided into seventeen chapters. The first half of the book describes the function of the heart with a clarity and accuracy utterly new to medicine. The second half lays out Harvey's theory concerning the blood vessels with careful logic and, as always, the support of detailed observations. Then came the revolution, but it was not a shock to anyone who had read the preceding chapters: "I am obliged to conclude," Harvey wrote with bland assurance, "that in animals the blood is driven round a circuit with an unceasing, circular sort of movement, that this is an activity or function of the heart which it carries out by virtue of its pulsation, and that in sum it constitutes the sole reason for that heart's pulsatile movement."[19]

De Motu Cordis inspired detractors to take up their pens in opposition to Harvey's theory, but their number was surprisingly small, considering the tension that had greeted earlier efforts to advance knowledge of the heart. Circulation was included in medical school lectures throughout most of Europe within two decades, a mere blink of an eye in a medical world that had formerly counted progress in terms of millennia. A contemporary pointed out that Dr. Harvey was "the only man, perhaps, that ever lived to see his owne Doctrine established in his life-time."[20] Harvey pursued further research in embryology, even as he continued to practice, sometimes traveling in the company of the king.

One case that attracted great interest in London was that of Thomas Parr, a farmer from a village in Shropshire. When Harvey's friend the earl of Arundel heard on a visit to the area that Parr had reached the wizened age of 152, he took an immediate interest in the old man and even arranged to bring him to London to meet King Charles. That was all it took. Within a few months, Old Parr was dead—done in, not by time, but by rich food and London air, according to William Harvey's subsequent autopsy. Parr's actual age has been doubted by modern writers,[21] but Harvey believed it. And he built a timeless reputation on objectivity.

The latter part of Harvey's life was filled with controversy and, at one point, utter ruination, but not because of his medical views. While that was a brawl that didn't quite materialize, a civil war did erupt in England in 1642, encompassing the king's good friend William Harvey in its dizzy and destructive path. Decidedly out of favor after the defeat and beheading of Charles I, Harvey lived quietly until the end of his own life in 1657. Long since a widower, he stayed during his last years with one or another of his wealthy merchant brothers.

The theory of blood circulation, as dramatic as it was, was no instant inspiration. No apple fell on Harvey's head, as the lore has it surrounding his countryman Isaac Newton. Harvey relied on the unending discipline of scientific observation. While he was very much a man of his times, his greatest strength lay in the fact that he had an abundant intellect, undistracted by imagination.

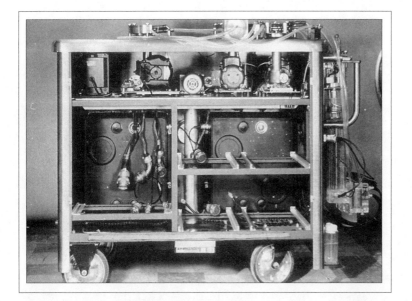

John H. Gibbon Jr.
LONG WAY TO BYPASS

After Charles Lindbergh flew across the Atlantic Ocean alone in 1927, he became such a celebrity that when he developed an interest in the possibility of organ replacement two years later, he was invited to the Rockefeller Institute to work with Dr. Alexis Carrel, a Nobel laureate eminent in the field of cell culture. Forty years later, Colonel Lindbergh told Dr. Clarence Dennis how it was that he came to start thinking about medical engineering: His wife Anne's sister had been diagnosed with a serious cardiac condition, one that her doctors claimed they could correct if only heart surgery were possible. It wasn't possible, though, because, as they explained to Lindbergh, so much blood gushed around the heart cavity that surgeons couldn't hope to see what they were doing. Dr. Dennis, himself a pioneer in the development of the heart-lung machine in the early 1950s, credited Lindbergh as the first person to think seriously about ways to temporarily replace the function of the heart and lung, so as to drain the heart cavity for surgery.

As preposterous as it seems for a pilot to be masquerading as a medical researcher, the fact is that Lindbergh brought to the nascent field of organ replacement exactly what it needed, which was practical engineering. If his character ultimately did not prove equal to the discipline required by medical research, at least he was, as ever, convenient as a symbol, a signpost of something new that was ready to attach itself to medicine.

In 1936, Carrel and Lindbergh demonstrated a new medical apparatus at a conference in Copenhagen. Called an artificial heart by the popular press, it was actually the very first step toward such a thing, designed only to keep one isolated organ (a thyroid, for example), supplied with enough blood and oxygen to maintain its vitality for short periods. Unfortunately, Dr. Carrel's influence over Charles Lindbergh soon expanded past medical matters, into theories regarding the doom of America's mingled nationalities. Within a year or two, Lindbergh's public activities in espousing similar views apparently interested him more than any start he'd made in medical research, which he set aside for good.

Independently of Charles Lindbergh, a young physician named John Gibbon Jr. was thinking out the principle of the heart-lung machine in 1931. But unlike Lindbergh, he would not quit, no matter how long it took to succeed.

Born in Philadelphia in 1903, Gibbon came from a long line of doctors, starting with his great-great-grandfather. He had the idea of becoming a poet, though, and after graduating from Princeton, he finally broke the news to his father, who was professor of surgery at the Jefferson Medical School in Philadelphia. John Sr. talked him into going into the family business instead.

John Jr., known as Jack, graduated from Jefferson Medical School in 1927. With an eye toward dividing his career between the operating room and the laboratory, he became a research fellow under Dr. Edward Churchill at the Massachusetts General Hospital in Boston.

Having learned in medical school the astounding things that a doctor could do, Gibbon handled a case in 1931 that demonstrated with blunt tragedy one thing that a doctor could not even hope to do. A young woman complaining of severe chest pain was diagnosed as having a blockage known as an embolus. Dr. Churchill knew just how to clear it, but there was one drawback. He could not proceed unless her heart stopped. Unfortunately, that is just what happened, so Churchill took advantage of the only chance left, opening her chest and clearing the blockage in a matter of minutes. By then, though, it was too late to revive her.[1]

Gibbon had been forced to stand by, little more than a witness, as the woman died but for a simple operation. Shaken by the experience, he didn't see why a machine couldn't temporarily perform the functions of the heart and lungs, so that a surgeon would have a "dry" chest cavity in which to operate. It was a great idea—and an utterly preposterous one in 1931.

It would also be preposterous to most of the medical world in 1950, when Gibbon was still working to perfect his heart-lung machine. In fact, he received so little encouragement during his long years of research that he practically hugged Dr. Dennis the first time he met him in 1946, as Dennis recalled, "with the comment that now there was someone else in the world who did not consider him an impossible dreamer."

Gibbon did have one thing going for him as he began full-time research on the heart-lung machine in 1934: his new wife, Mary ("Maly") Hopkinson, had been Dr. Churchill's research assistant, and she was as interested in the idea of the machine as he was. Maly had dropped out of Bryn Mawr College a few years earlier in order to study piano in Paris; while there, she stayed with her cousin Frances Eliot and her husband, Frank Fremont-Smith. A physician, Fremont-Smith would later head the Josiah Macy Jr. Foundation. Maly was so engrossed by the medical discussions held each evening in their home that she took a course upon her return to Boston and qualified as a research assistant.[2] During the 1930s, she and Gibbon made an efficient team, and a resourceful one. "The Federal Government," Gibbon later recalled, "was not then pouring out hundreds of millions of dollars to doctors to perform research. Harvard provided my fellowship and the Massachusetts General Hospital provided the laboratory. I bought an air pump in a second-hand shop down in East Boston for a few dollars . . . Valves were made from solid rubber corks with the small end cut transversely."[3]

The challenge in creating the machine did not lay in replicating the pumping action of the heart, which was fairly simple, but in taking over for the lungs.[4] The iron lung, which had been developed at Harvard Medical School in 1929, regulated pressure and gases to assist an ailing lung; the heart-lung machine Gibbon had in mind would have to do much more, completely replacing the patient's lungs by assuming their two primary functions: putting oxygen into the blood and taking carbon dioxide out. Learning to oxygenate the blood was hard enough, but handling blood without damaging cells and other components was a continual problem.

In 1934, the Gibbons proved that they were on the right track, keeping a cat alive for a few minutes with a rudimentary heart-lung machine they made in their Boston lab. By the late 1930s, the Gibbons had moved back to Philadelphia, where Jack bought more time for the heart-lung machine with a fellowship at the University of Pennsylvania School of Medicine. The Josiah Macy Jr. Foundation also provided funding.

In 1939, Jack and Maly were able to demonstrate the basic viability of the heart-lung system by maintaining the life of a cat for up to 20 minutes and, what is more, returning it to its own pulmonary system. For the first time, a machine had temporarily assumed the function of the heart and lungs in an animal. The system consisted of two pumps, one to draw the blood from the vein and one to send it back to an artery, with a revolving drum in between, to spread the blood over an oxygenating film. Most observers still had doubts about the machine, however. A cat is an animal that requires very little oxygen, even for its size. Time and again, elders in the medical community advised Jack Gibbon to find a less radical course of research, telling him that even if he failed, it would be better for his career to stay closer to the pack. With every year that he worked on the heart-lung machine, he was risking more and more of his future. But it isn't hard to fathom what kept the Gibbons working on a machine that no one else considered truly viable. "If the flow of blood through the heart and lungs could be safely stopped for 30 minutes," Jack Gibbon wrote in 1939, "it is conceivable that a new field of cardiac surgery might be developed."[5]

With the United States' entry into World War II, however, John Gibbon set his research aside. He packed his inventions away and left to serve with the Army in the South Pacific. In addition to treating soldiers, he became the chess champion of a large section of the Pacific Theater. After returning in 1945, he became a professor at Jefferson Medical School in Philadelphia. And without missing a beat, he returned as well to the development of the heart-lung machine. However, he did not have the same outlook as before the war. He had come to realize that he could not complete the project and solve the problems with oxygenation by working on his own. Maly Gibbon, who had been instrumental in the early development of the machine, was no longer available for research; she was busy with their five children.

Gibbon was aware that he needed help in the form of expert engineers. On hearing of the problem, one of his colleagues mentioned that a freshman in the medical school, a former aviator, had invented a machine for transcribing music and had worked with International Business Machines on the idea. Gibbon contacted the student and asked him if he thought IBM would be interested in cooperating on a heart-lung machine. "The student thought it quite likely," Gibbon later recalled, and during the Christmas vacation of 1946,[6] he made a trip to the IBM Building in New York. He was taken almost immediately to see the chairman, Thomas J. Watson Sr., who had taken charge of IBM as a collection of bankrupt companies in 1914. Watson was an icon of American business in the 1940s, a man who had built his reputation on equal parts efficiency and humanity. Almost thirty years later, Gibbon recalled the day:

I shall never forget the first time I met Mr. Watson at his office in New York City. He came into the anteroom where I sat, carrying reprints of my publications. He shook my hand

and sat down beside me. He said the idea [of a heart-lung machine] was interesting and asked what he could do to help. I remember replying rather bluntly that I did not want him to make any money from the idea, nor did I wish to make any money from it. He brushed my comments aside with a wave of his hand and said, 'Don't worry about that.' . . . From that time on we not only had engineering help always available, but IBM paid the entire cost of constructing the various machines with which we carried on the work for the next seven years.[7]

During World War II, the dominant nations had gathered scientists into veritable armies of invention that not only changed the means of war with each week that went by but left their particular fields littered with new materials, methods, theories, and mechanisms. In the aftermath, engineers and scientists themselves were part of a formula, newly apparent: that minds plus money could equal anything at all.

In the new environment, the U.S. Public Health Service allotted its first grants for research in 1949, directing about $29,000 (a respectable 4 percent of its overall budget) to Gibbon for the development of a heart-lung machine. Gibbon was no longer made to feel anything like an impossible dreamer. Even as Thomas Watson had become convinced of the need for an artificial replacement for the heart, so had many other people: In the late 1940s, heart disease was by far the leading cause of death in the United States. Four million people had a serious heart condition; six hundred thousand of them died each year. So desperate was the need for some way to operate that the breakthrough of 1948 was a new technique by which the surgeon connected a scalpel to the tip of one finger and operated by touch. Others made do with major surgery of a harrowingly minor sort: tying off the blood vessels to drain the heart cavity for about three minutes. That would not be long enough to cause brain damage: It was surgery against the clock, and it wouldn't suit more than a small percentage of cases (or surgeons). A third means of rudimentary heart surgery lay in experiments with cross-transfusions—letting the heart of a healthy person pump blood for both himself and the patient undergoing corrective surgery. None of that was good enough. The development of a machine to make corrective surgery possible was the first priority for about a half-dozen teams working in the U.S. John Gibbon may have been the first, but he was no longer alone in the field.

Even while Watson was loaning engineers from IBM to work with Gibbon on the oxygenating drum in his heart-lung system, Charles E. Wilson was listening to a presentation by a Detroit surgeon named Forest Dodrill, who had made sketches for his own heart-lung machine and needed help in realizing them. Wilson was chairman of both the Michigan State Heart Association and the General Motors Corporation. Midway through the meeting, he called in several of GM's research engineers. "We have pumped oil, gasoline, water, and other fluids one way or another in our business. It seems only logical we should try to pump blood," said one of them, as Wilson committed GM to the project.

At about the same time, Dr. Dennis at the University of Minnesota began what he later called "a methodical evaluation of a series of configurations" of heart-lung machines. He was soon making a system according to designs he originated with colleagues at the university. By 1950, teams at other institutions were in the race—which is what it had become. In part, it was a race against the lack of a heart-lung machine. But it was also a race for glory, if not for reasons of ego, then for the practical fact that there was surely grant money waiting across the finish line. (Gibbon and IBM had already agreed to reassign any profits they might make to further research. General Motors and Forest Dodrill's team had a similar arrangement.

At each institution, dogs or cats were used for experiments, and the number of minutes that one could be sustained on a heart-lung machine became the tally of the race. Gibbon made headlines in

1949 when one of his cats survived for forty-six minutes. In Michigan, a total of eighty-four dogs underwent actual heart operations, beginning to end, and none of them died. In Minnesota, Dr. Dennis had his heart-lung machines sustaining dogs for almost three hours. But at some point, the heart-lung machine was going to have to be tried on a human being.

Dr. Willem Kolff, who was refining his artificial kidney at the same time, wasn't daunted by the prospect of human trials. "If one of 1,000 patients treated with an artificial organ or device dies," he wrote, "the press has a heyday, there is pandemonium. If 100,000 people die because a device that could have saved them is not applied, no one says a word."

In 1951, a six-year-old girl arrived at the University of Minnesota hospital with blue skin and irregular breathing. An exploratory operation proved her doctors' suspicions that there was a hole in a wall in her heart. It could have been stitched, except for the old problem of access to the heart cavity. A heart-lung machine could be put to use, except that Dr. Dennis's apparatus was configured for use with dogs. There wasn't any other hope for the girl, though, and so in a matter of days the machine was prepared for its first trial with a human patient. The operation took place, but the girl died after forty minutes from loss of blood. Her death would have been inevitable without the attempt at surgery, but that didn't necessarily comfort the family, or the doctors.

With the new equipment ready but not yet certain, the easiest route was to use it on cases that were otherwise hopeless—then no one could blame the doctors for failure. Safe public relations is not necessarily smart science, though. The heart-lung machine actually needed patients with relatively minor problems and the courage to try a technology regarded as radical at the time.

In 1952, a man arrived at Harper Hospital in Detroit with heart damage left by rheumatic fever. He was forty-one, and fit the necessary profile for an experimental case: He was relatively healthy, other than the fact that his heart trouble was degenerating toward a fatal conclusion. The machine developed by GM's engineers and Dr. Dodrill's team of doctors was capable of pumping blood; the lung function wasn't ready, but it wasn't necessary in this case. Surgeons used the artificial heart to pump for the left side of the man's heart, and that allowed them to see the damage and the repair as they made it. For the patient, the operation was the beginning of a new life. For the medical world, it was no less promising.

In May of 1953, Gibbon, working at the Jefferson Medical College in Philadelphia, took in a case that was similar to that of the little girl in Minnesota: The patient was a college freshman with a hole in the wall of her heart, between the auricles. Her heart condition was certainly serious, but she was still in good shape otherwise. Gibbon explained to her that he could close the hole in her heart with the use of the heart-lung machine.

Gibbon's initial revolving drum design had been refined by IBM to incorporate a grid pattern on stationary metal plates that created just enough turbulence to oxygenate the blood, but not so much, as in the case of the drum, as to damage cells. The patient, Cecilia Bavolek, agreed to the operation, which took place on May 6, 1953. For forty-five minutes, her most vital systems were connected to the heart-lung machine. More important, for twenty-seven minutes, her heart and lungs stopped entirely while the machine kept her alive.[8]

Dr. Gibbon had crossed the finish line he had first spotted in 1931, but the tension weighed heavily on him. "I think it was the only surgical operation," he wrote, "that I have ever performed for which I did not write or dictate the operative procedures and findings myself . . . I suppose that I did not want to relive the tension and emotional excitement by again recalling the details."[9]

For Bavolek, the ending was entirely happy. She was home within two weeks of open-heart surgery and went on to a healthy life. *Time* magazine pointed out in its report of the pioneering operation that Gibbon had been working on the heart-lung machine since before his patient was even born. After the initial success, though, Gibbon's design revealed flaws: After five operations, Bavolek was the only patient to survive implementation of the heart-lung machine. While other teams brought different versions of the heart-lung machine into use, Dr. John Kirklin at the Mayo Clinic picked up on Gibbon's design in 1955 and improved it for use on human patients.

Dr. Gibbon left the field to others after performing the first bypass heart operation, now often known simply as the "May 6 operation." Emotion had carried him through twenty-two years of uncertainty to that moment. Gibbon's belief, bordering on passion, had also propelled the wider field, once others started developing heart-lung machines. Having changed the surgical world, however, John Gibbon felt uncomfortable about his role. "Several years later," he wrote in 1970, referring to the aftermath of the May 6 operation, "when heart-lung machines were in general use throughout the world, I remember my dislike of opening a surgical journal and finding it full of articles on open heart surgery, thinking, I suppose, that I had opened some kind of Pandora's box."[10] That attitude would be responsible for a sad coda to Gibbon's life.

After Gibbon retired in 1967, he and Maly enjoyed a pleasant life on their farm in Pennsylvania. He came to recognize the overwhelmingly positive effect of his heart-lung machine, saying in a speech that it gave him great satisfaction to know that bypass operations were being performed on a daily basis all over the world. Yet in the early 1970s, Gibbon himself developed signs of heart trouble: a mild heart attack followed by angina. His close friend, Dr. Harris Schumacker, suggested time and again that he have a coronary arteriogram. "He knew full well," Schumacker wrote, "that there was a reasonably good possibility that this test would reveal a situation amenable either to a balloon dilatation or an operative aortic-coronary bypass procedure, and could in this way be assured of an extended period of enjoyable, active life. He didn't respond to my suggestions, though."[11]

Gibbon seemed reluctant to undergo the very bypass surgery

that he had pioneered—and that had already saved millions of other people. John H. Gibbon Jr. died of a heart attack in 1973, while playing tennis.

The race was far more important to him than the finish. He liked to remember the occasion in 1934 when he and Maly were first able to keep a cat alive, though its heart was stopped, using the equipment they'd made themselves. "I will never forget," he wrote in 1972, "the day when we were able to screw the clamp down all the way, completely occluding the pulmonary artery, with the extracorporeal blood circuit in operation and with no change in the animal's blood pressure. My wife and I threw our arms around each other and danced around the laboratory laughing and shouting hooray. . . nothing in my life has duplicated the ecstacy and joy of that dance with Mary around the laboratory of the old Bulfinch building in the Massachusetts General Hospital twenty-eight years ago."[12]

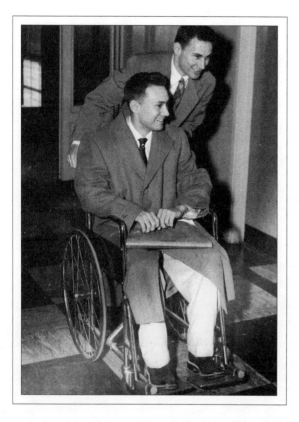

Joseph E. Murray and
John P. Merrill
A Bit of Life

A kidney performs about a half-dozen functions, but the one that becomes a matter of life and death very quickly is the removal of waste and excess water from the bloodstream. People with kidney failure become comatose because they are poisoning themselves, as unhealthy substances collect more and more densely in their systems. A healthy kidney keeps the bloodstream clean through the action of glomeruli, tufts of very fine blood vessels called capillaries, of which there are about a million in a kidney.

The walls of the glomeruli are sieves, pocked with holes that are big enough to let molecules of water and waste (known as urea) slip through, but too small to let any vital cells or matter out. Over the course of the entire process, elements carried by the blood passes first one way and then the other through the holes, but by the time the blood is on its way out of the kidney, vital chemical balances have been restored.

A kidney is an ingenious piece of engineering, renewing itself even as it conditions the blood. Yet it has a rather humble air, if a personality could be ascribed to a lopsided bit of pulp. The kidneys go along very quietly. No emotional upheaval has ever been blamed on a kidney, as with the liver, spleen, and, of course, the heart; the Renaissance poets seem to have ignored it entirely.

It was the kidney, however, that gave rise to a new field, and more important, to a new medical philosophy, by validating the whole idea of transplantation. Less complex than some organs, less delicate than others, yet just as crucial as any of them, it offered a starting point. Surgeons on the outermost edge of hope after World War II could only imagine replacing a malfunctioning kidney, conferring about it in small groups of believers. Where to find the new organ was one of the first problems they faced. Another was ensuring that it would be accepted by the recipient's body after the great miracle, the transplantation, was over. Teams of doctors in America and France were bearing down on research and collecting some strands of confidence in the early 1950s, yet those two major problems remained.

In late October 1954, a young man named Richard Herrick was admitted to Peter Bent Brigham Hospital in Boston. His kidneys were failing and his blood was loaded with so many toxins that it could no longer absorb impurities from the cells in his other systems. Given only a few weeks to live, he was placed under observation by Dr. Joseph E. Murray and Dr. John P. Merrill, coleaders of a team assigned to conduct research into the possibility of kidney transplantation. Normally, a person in Herrick's condition had no chance of survival, but his case was unique in one important respect that made it interesting to the doctors at Brigham Hospital. He had an identical twin.

The emaciated Herrick was suffering from congestive heart failure, high blood pressure, and incoherence bordering on insanity, all due to the deterioration of his kidneys.[1] Like 20,000 other doomed patients in the U.S., he needed a new kidney. Murray and Merrill were his last hope, but they had never performed a kidney transplant. No one had, with any success.

The first kidney transplants were attempted in 1902 and the decade that followed by doctors using a strangely haphazard approach to donor selection: a dog's kidney implanted in a goat, a pig's in a human, an infant's kidney (from a baby who died soon after at birth) in a baboon, and so forth. If the various experimenters, working in

France and Germany, were more zealous than methodical, it was because they felt newly empowered by the work of Alexis Carrel, a Frenchman who was later a Nobel Prize winner and, still later, an infamous Nazi sympathizer. In 1902, Carrel announced new techniques for suturing blood vessels, making surgeons feel sure that they could attach organs, starting with kidneys, to practically anything more animated than a stuffed animal. Much later, looking back on those early trials, the English surgeon Roy Yorke Calne wrote, "The distinction between failures due to technical faults and those due to biological factors have been slowly recognized."[2]

For almost forty years, very little was done in transplant research, mostly because, as Calne indicated, surgeons could not be certain whether the hurdle ultimately lay with their operating methods (technical faults) or with the fact that a living body wouldn't want a replacement kidney, no matter how beautifully crafted into place (biological factors). In 1946, though, a surgeon at Boston's Brigham Hospital, Dr. David Hume, was working feverishly to save a patient with kidney failure and tried a procedure that might be considered a "halfway" transplant. He attached a kidney to the vessels in a patient's arm. It probably didn't look very pretty, but it did work for a few days, until the body began to reject it. In that interim, however, the patient's own kidney function returned, and so the operation was considered a success.[3] The department chiefs at Brigham were impressed enough to set a high priority on research into kidney transplantation, assigning Dr. Hume, Dr. Merrill, and, later, Dr. Murray to explore the possibilities.

John Merrill, who was trained in internal medicine, was only thirty years old in 1947, but he had already had one brush with history, as the Army Air Corps flight surgeon for the crew of the *Enola Gay*, which dropped an atomic bomb on Hiroshima, in 1945.[4] Returning to his alma mater, Harvard Medical School, after the war, Merrill made a specialty of studying kidney disease. In 1951, he and Dr. Hume undertook nine more of those halfway transplants (known as allografts), in which they attached a replacement kidney to the thigh of a patient whose own kidneys were failing. In each instance, the organ was ultimately rejected, though in one case it lasted for six months.

In 1952, John Merrill took a one-year sabbatical at the Necker Hospital in Paris, where important work in the field of kidney transplantation was already being done. While he was there, a sixteen-year-old carpenter was admitted with a ruptured right kidney, suffered when he fell off a scaffold. It seemed at first to be a matter of no real consequence. Most people have two kidneys, though both aren't necessary. One person in a thousand, on average, is born with only a single kidney, and is usually never even aware of it.

The carpenter was rushed into surgery to remove the damaged kidney. When the surgeons opened him up, they found that the poor young man was that one in a thousand: He had been born with only one kidney. He was suddenly in the midst of a crisis. Dialysis, the process of cleansing the blood through a mechanical apparatus, was still a fairly new option in 1952. It could keep the youth alive temporarily, but his condition was bound to deteriorate. The patient's mother, with her rudimentary understanding of physiology, begged the doctors to take one of her kidneys and give it to her son.

The usual specter of organ rejection loomed over the prospect of having the mother serve as a kidney donor, yet there was some reason to think the idea held promise. By 1952, there were two approaches to the goal of discouraging rejection (the body's natural inclination to attack and destroy foreign organisms). The first was based on genetics: As specimens, some people, of course, are more alike than others. That is true in terms of broad characteristics, such as blood type, as well as other factors continuing down to the most specific, the DNA structure. Successful experiments with skin grafts between identical twins had proven in 1950–51 that the body, even while on guard against unfriendly intrusions, would accommodate matching organs (skin being an organ, after all). The theory that emerged from that research held that as long as the body doesn't perceive a transplanted organ as being "foreign," it won't attack it.

If that first theory focused on the body's will to reject organs, the second addressed its ability to do so. It suggested that methods might be found to weaken the body's immune system, giving the transplanted kidney a chance to establish itself. Researchers in France and the U.S. found a promising method to accomplish just that by using radiation in advance of an operation to suppress the immune response. Anyway, it worked with rabbits.

The doctors at Necker Hospital had some confidence in the radiation technique, but never enough to make them want to chance a human transplantation experiment. The carpenter's case offered a reason to reconsider. Tests revealed a "close immunologic relationship between mother and son," which seemed to allay the genetic concerns regarding rejection. Still, the French team, led by Dr. Jean Hamburger, fretted. Their convictions discouraged them from doing anything that might jeopardize the patient—or, in this case, the mother-donor. "We might never have gone on to attempt the procedure in man but for the influence of John P. Merrill," Hamburger wrote twenty years later.

He had come to spend a sabbatical year in Paris and we soon fell under the spell of this patrician Bostonian with the inquiring mind, who was firmly convinced that desperate diseases called for daring remedies. One day, during a discussion on the new and difficult ethical problems of kidney transplantation in man, he said, "Your fears and hesitant attitude seem wrong to me. Think of all the patients who may die because you have not had the courage to do what was necessary to add to our knowledge and open the way to new methods of treatment."[5]

The operation went ahead, and the carpenter received one of his mother's kidneys. For three weeks he rallied, but that was all that the combined effect of radiation and a "close" genetic match offered to him. When his body ultimately rejected the kidney, he died. However, his mother got at least the first part of her wish: Everything possible had been done for her son. And, as Merrill had suggested, "real knowledge" had been added to advance the possibility of organ replacement.

In 1953, Richard Herrick was just another twenty-four-year-old, about to be discharged from the Coast Guard. However, during a routine physical in Chicago, where he was stationed, his blood pressure was found to be unusually high.[6] With further tests, doctors found that he had glomerulonephritis, or inflammation of the kidney.[7] The cause was not known, though it may have been triggered by an infection picked up somewhere. Herrick had grown up in comfortable circumstances on a farm outside of Boston, and so when his condition deteriorated, he was transferred to the Public Health Service Hospital in Brighton, Mass. His parents had long since died, but his two brothers and his sister visited him frequently, and were shocked to see him losing more weight and color by the day. Their grandfather, a general practitioner, said that there was no cure for the condition and no hope for Richard.[8]

The doctor handling Herrick's daily care at the hospital was a young intern named David C. Miller. One day while the family was visiting, Miller was in the room. "So," recalled Ronald Herrick, the patient's twin brother, "my older brother Van said to the doctor, 'Too bad I couldn't give him one of my kidneys.' The doctor said, 'Well, that's a nice idea, but it's impossible.' "[9] A moment later, however, Dr. Miller remembered reading about transplantation research at Brigham Hospital, in which genetic matching was a primary concern. He contacted the research team at the hospital and suggested that "since the patient has a twin brother, Ronald . . . the possibility of homotransplantation [surgery involving two humans] should be considered."[10]

By the time Richard Herrick reached Brigham on October 26, 1954, he was a very sick man. Practically every bodily system was affected by his kidney failure. His heart was congested, his skin was sallow, his digestion was completely chaotic, and worst of all he was psychotic, cursing madly and going so far as to bite a nurse at one point. That was no more typical of the real Richard Herrick than was the fact that the former sailor barely had the strength to stand up.

Dr. Merrill and Dr. J. Hartwell Harrison, a urologist, oversaw treatment of Herrick's immediate problems through a program that included dialysis. Within days, his mental balance returned, and so did a measure of his former good health. Major issues, however, remained. Many of them were left to Dr. Murray, who had by then replaced David Hume as the lead surgeon on the transplantation team. Unfortunately, with the outbreak of the Korean War, Hume had been called into the Army medical corps, and he was to miss the dramatic advances in the field he had done so much to launch.

Joseph Murray was raised near Boston and knew from his earliest years that he wanted to be a surgeon. Medicine didn't run in his family, though: His father was a lawyer and his mother was active in politics, attending every Democratic National Convention from 1920 to 1976. A year after graduating from Harvard Medical School in 1943, Dr. Murray was drafted into the Army. Although World War II was winding down, he was kept all too busy at an Army hospital in Pennsylvania, treating badly disfigured GIs through reconstructive surgery. In 1947, he returned to Boston and the Brigham Hospital, where he not only continued to develop his skills as a plastic surgeon, but also became involved in the ongoing transplantation research.

Two weeks after Herrick was admitted late in 1954, Dr. Murray initiated testing to confirm the genetic compatibility of the patient and his brother, Ronald. Just because they were twins and looked about the same didn't make them identical for purposes of the transplantation experiment. Murray looked at their blood chemistry and made successful skin grafts, but he didn't stop there. "I called the police down at the local station and told them what we were going to do," he recalled, "and could they do some fingerprinting, because the fingerprints had to be within a certain pattern of similarity." The fingerprints passed, as did all the twins' other results.

With the Herrick case, the biological factor would be removed from kidney transplantation: As long as the operation was performed correctly, the transplanted kidney wouldn't be rejected, according to accepted knowledge of the time. It was a rare opportunity to save a patient's life and, at the same time, test the very basis of that knowledge in the field of transplantation. Dr. Merrill and Dr. Harrison would perform the operation on Ronald Herrick, the healthy twin, to remove his left kidney. Dr. Murray, the expert surgeon, would handle the transplantation itself, placing the donated organ into Richard Herrick's system.

Since Richard's two ailing kidneys were to remain in place for the time being, Murray had to think through a very basic part of his plan: where to fit the extra kidney. He chose a space in the abdomen that would require only a little crowding against the large intestine.

One last question remained, and it rested with Ronald Herrick: He had to decide whether or not to go through with the operation. On several occasions, Murray, Merrill, and Harrison met with the Herrick family to explain the procedure and answer questions as they arose. Naturally, Ronald wanted to know whether he could expect any problems living with just one kidney; as he was told, a person isn't any better off with two kidneys than with one, except in the unlikely event of an injury or cancer of the kidney. The more common renal diseases (as with Richard's infection) run the same course whether a person has one kidney or two.[11]

"They left it up to me to decide," Ronald later said, speaking of both his family and the team at Brigham. "I was the one who was going to do it; they weren't going to make the decision for me."[12] Ronald loved his brother, and without much vacillation, he decided to go ahead with the transplant, which was then scheduled for December 23. He did have one moment of panic on the morning of the operation, though. Having grown to trust Dr. Harrison in particular, he raised a ruckus when he somehow got the idea that an intern would perform the operation. Immediately, he was assured that Harrison, along with Merrill, would be his surgeons. The nephrectomy—the removal of Ronald's healthy kidney—was the less worrisome operation, though.

Just as countless shoeboxes rattling with gears and levers testify to the fact that dismantling a clock is never as daunting as putting it back together, connecting the sensitive vessels in a kidney transplantation requires coordination and expertise of the highest order. It also calls for experience of a sort that no one had in 1954. Joseph Murray was well aware of that fact as he drove toward the hospital early on the day of the operation. "I won't say I offered any special prayers for the success of the Herrick transplant," he wrote. "All I know is that I drove into Boston on the morning of the operation determined to do the very best work possible."[13]

The operation began at 8:15 A.M., when Murray prepared Herrick to receive a new kidney. Timing was of the essence. At 9:50, he was ready for the new kidney, and only three minutes later, Dr. Merrill carried it in, very carefully, from an adjoining operation room.

At 11:15, Murray finished connecting the new kidney to Richard Herrick's blood vessels. The kidney had been without blood flow for an hour and twenty-two minutes. Possible damage from the lack of circulating blood had been a major concern of the surgical team. However, when Murray looked down into the cavity in Herrick's abdomen at 11:15, he couldn't help being pleased. At that moment, according to a later report, "The entire kidney became turgid and pink immediately on release of the arterial clamp. . . It lay rather neatly in its new site." Best of all, as the report noted, "There was a brisk flow of urine . . . from the ureteral catheter."[14]

It worked.

Ronald Herrick, the donor, went home from the hospital within two weeks, none the worse for wear. Five weeks after the operation, Richard Herrick was discharged too, almost fully recovered. And his old charms must have returned by then; he soon became engaged to his recovery-room nurse.

The operation had been covered in the Boston papers, but it didn't become international news until the following year. By then, Richard Herrick was living a normal life, filled with wedding talk, classes in television engineering and a host of other, rather unremarkable plans for the future.[15] And that was just what made it remarkable. A man whose kidneys had failed was alive and well—an epochal change in the history of internal medicine. Herrick had not been cured, the age-old goal of medicine. He had not even been repaired, the commonplace goal of surgery. Richard Herrick had been rebuilt.

As the first transplant of a major organ from one person to another, the operation in Boston made a striking statement about medicine, as well as the world beyond. Up to that point, humans viewed themselves against the backdrop of medicine only in individual terms. A being—the usual measurement of human existence—was always expressed in the singular form. With transplantation, though, life or some crucial component of it passed from one individual to another. If humans were regarded from afar and not on a sentimental basis, it might be presumed that transplantation had more to do with the health of the species (and ultimately its propagation) than of those specific names it kept out of the obituary pages.

Doctors were, as ever, in the business of treating individuals after the advent of transplantation, but the medicine they had in their power to give was, for the first time, taken from neither the chemical world nor the natural one, but from the human kingdom. They were doling out something taken, in the broadest sense, from the whole race for the whole race. That new pursuit, grown commonplace today, of looking to the human body—that is, other people's human bodies—as the fount of new medicines, started with the first successful kidney transplant, in Boston on December 23, 1954.

At the time, skeptics pointed out that the Herrick operation was a very great breakthrough—in the treatment of identical twins. However, doctors in Boston and in France continued their efforts, making advances that moved transplantation one step at a time beyond the province of identical twins. Richard Herrick lived an active life for eight years after his operation, but ultimately, the glomerulonephritis that had affected his own kidneys returned, though they had been removed within months of the transplant. He died in 1962.

John Merrill and Joseph Murray both remained active in the field that grew in the wake of the Herrick operation. Merrill concentrated on his primary interest in nephrology, or the study of diseases of the kidney. He retired in the early 1980s and tragically drowned after falling off a sailboat in the Bahamas in 1984. Through the years, Murray stayed closer to research in organ replacement, receiving the Nobel Prize for Medicine in 1990 for his leadership in making kidney transplantation a viable reality.

Starting in the mid-1960s with the introduction of immunosuppressant drugs, kidney transplants became more and more common.[16] By the 1980s, better drugs and improved operative techniques vastly increased the number of patients eligible for transplant surgery, but they soon outstripped the number of organs available. As of 2003, there were 80,000 Americans in need of a kidney transplant, according to the National Kidney Foundation.[17] In a good year, 14,000 kidneys become available.[18] Meanwhile, 6,200 people will have died on the waiting list.[19] Philosophical issues related to organ transplant have exploded into far more immediate concerns, as people who can't wait their turn advertise for live donors or turn to illegal schemes that pay live donors, especially in impoverished regions of the world, to give up one kidney. The trade in organs has at times sunk to practices even more grisly than that, with the executions of convicts in China delayed for the sake of paying customers who want to harvest the organs. The kidneys are removed at the hospital; the prisoner dies while still under anesthetic.[20]

By 2002, the number of kidneys derived from live donors had surpassed the number taken from cadavers at many transplantation centers.[21] The majority of live donors in the U.S. are relatives or acquaintances of the patient. Even for the small number of live donors who donate one of their kidneys to a stranger, it is an act of love in some sense of the word. Yet the shortage remains. For reasons that are more personal than those on nearly any other issue, people who would gladly give up a kidney while alive can't bring themselves to do it in anticipation of death. Perhaps the instinct to regard the body as a personal fortress against death will have to change, but something stops the majority of people from consigning their organs—some part of the mystery that is shrouded by the body and its parts.

That reluctance is, if nothing else, an individual act. While it undoubtedly constrains the rate of transplantation, as well as the hopes of those awaiting operations, it is only a reminder that the metamorphosis started by the first kidney transplant is not yet fifty years old. It is possible that people still don't fully understand what transplantation means, not even those who have worked within the field for decades.

ENDNOTES

I. Understanding the Body

The Art of Medicine

1. M. H. Spielman, *Iconography of Andreas Vesalius,* (London: J. Bale and Danielsson, 1925), p. xiii

2. Roland H. Bainton, "Changing Ideas and ideals in the Sixteenth Century, *Journal of Modern History,* vol. 8, no. 4, Dec. 1936, p. 422

3. C. S. Sherrington, *Endeavor of Jean Fernel,* excerpted in John Farquhar Fulton, *Vesalius Four Centuries Later* (Lawrenceville: Univ. Of Kansas, 1950), p. 8

4. Dr. James J. Walsh, "Debt of Medical Science to the Early Printers" *Scientific Monthly,* vol. 18, no. 2, Feb. 1924, p. 185

5. Walsh, "Debt of Medical Science to the Early Printers" p. 182

6. Charles Singer, *A Short History of Anatomy* (New York: Dover, 1957), p. 73

7. J. B. DeC. M. Saunders and Charles D. O'Malley, "The Preparation of the Human Skeleton by Andreas Vesalius of Brussels," *Bulletin of Medical History,* vol. 20, no. 1, June 1946, p. 434

8. Singer, *A Short History of Anatomy,* p. 75

9. Spielman, *Iconography of Andreas Vesalius,* p. xiv

10. Reinerus Solenander, letter dated May 1566, reprinted in Gregory Zilboorg, "Psychological Sidelights on Andreas Vesalius," *Bulletin of the History of Medicine,* vol. 14, no. 5, Dec. 1943, p. 564

11. Gregory Zilboorg, "Psychological Sidelights on Andreas Vesalius," *Bulletin of the History of Medicine,* vol. 14, no. 5, Dec., 1943, p. 564

12. Singer, *A Short History of Anatomy,* p. 114; Encyclopedia of the Scientific Revolution, p. 666

13. John Farquhar Fulton, *Vesalius Four Centuries Later,* (Lawrenceville: Univ. of Kansas), p. 10

14. Giorgio Vasari, *Le Vite de piu eccellenti pittori, scultori, e architettori,* translated and excerpted in R. Joseph Petrucelli II, "Giorgio Vasari's Attribution of the Vesalian Illustrations to Jan Stephan of Calcar: A Further Examination," *Bulletin of the History of Medicine,* vol. 45, no. 1, Jan–Feb, 1971, p. 35

15. W. M. Ivins Jr., "What About the 'Fabrica' of Vesalius?" in Samuel W. Lambert, editor, *Three Vesalian Essays to Accompany the Icones Anatomicae of 1934* (New York: Macmillan, 1952), pp. 96–7

16. Singer, *A Short History of Anatomy,* p. 111

Endnotes

17. Fulton, *Vesalius Four Centuries Later,* p. 17
18. "Metellus," letter dated 1565, trans. By Dr. C. D. O'Malley, reprinted in Fulton, p. 12–13
19. Singer, *A Short History of Anatomy,* p. 111

A Peculiar Light

1. Tamar Nordenberg, "The Picture of Health," *FDA Consumer,* vol. 33, no, 1, p. 10
2. Benedict Carey, "A Doctor's Bedside Manner is Great, but People Find Comfort in Technology," *Los Angeles Times,* June 25, 2001, p. S3
3. Ira B. Wilson MD, Kim Dukes MA, Sheldon Greenfield, MD, Sherrie Kaplan MPH, Bruce Hellman MD, "Patients' Role in the Use of Radiology Testing," *Archives of Internal Medicine,* vol. 161, Jan. 22, 2001, p. 261
4. Mary Batten, *Discovery by Chance,* (Chicago: Funk and Wagnalls, 1968), p. 123
5. Dr. Francis Carter Wood, "Marie Curie—Her Life Work," *Scientific Monthly,* vol. 46, no. 4, April, 1938, p. 378
6. Forest Ray Moulton and Justus J. Schifferes, *Autobiography of Science* (Garden City, N.Y.: Doubleday & Co., 1960), p. 484
7. George Sarton, "The Discovery of X-rays," *Isis,* vol. 26, no. 2, Mar. 1937, p. 352
8. Dr. Otto Glasser, *Dr. Wilhelm C. Röntgen* (Springfield, Ill.: Charles C. Thomas, 1945), p. 26
9. George I. Manes, M.D. "The Discovery of X-ray," *Isis,* vol. 47, no. 3, Sept, 1956, p. 237
10. W. Robert Nitske, *The Life of Wilhelm Conrad Röntgen,* (Tucson: Univ. of Arizona, 1971), p. 94
11. Dr. Otto Glasser, "The Life of Wilhelm Conrad Röntgen as Revealed in his Letters," *Scientific Monthly,* vol. 45, no. 3, Sept. 1937, p. 196
12. Glasser, "The Life of Wilhelm Conrad Röntgen as Revealed in his Letters,", p. 196; minor editorial changes were made to the translation for this book
13. Glasser, *Dr. Wilhelm C. Röntgen* (Springfield, Ill.: Charles C. Thomas, 1945), p. 57
14. Sarton, "The Discovery of X-rays," p. 356
15. Manes. "The Discovery of X-ray," p. 237
16. Wood, "Marie Curie," p. 380
17. Helen Clapesattle, *The Doctors Mayo,* (Minneapolis: Univ. Of Minnesota, 1941), p. 366
18. Loretta Boyd, J. Patrick O'Leary, "Roentgen and his Ray: An Early Impact on Modern Medicine," *American Surgeon,* vol. 65, no. 3, Mar. 1999, p. 293
19. "Dr. John Spence Dies; Was Martyr to X-Ray," *New York Times,* Mar. 16, 1930, p. 30
20. "Martyr of Science; Doctor's Arm Lost in X-Ray Work," *London Daily Mail,* February 17, 1908, p. 5
21. Glasser, "The Life of Wilhelm Conrad Röntgen as Revealed in his Letters," p. 198

Picture of Youth

1. J.M. Forrester, "Using oneself as one's only experimental subject," *Lancet,* vol. 336, Sept. 29, 1990, p. 798

2. Marilyn Chase, "French AIDS Researcher in Storm's Center," *Wall Street Journal,* June 8, 1987, p. 1

3. Renate Forssmann-Falck M.D., "Werner Forssmann: A Pioneer of Cardiology," *American Journal of Cardiology,* vol. 79, Mar. 1, 1997, p. 651

4. Werner Forssmann, *Experiments on Myself* (New York: St. Martin's, 1972), p. 21

5. Forssmann, *Experiments on Myself,* p. 29

6. Forssmann, *Experiments on Myself,* p. 77

7. Forssmann, *Experiments on Myself,* p. 81

8. Dickinson W. Richards, "Right Heart Catheterization," *Science,* vol. 125, no. 3259, June 14, 1957, p. 1181

9. Dr. Werner Forssmann, "Die Sondierung des Rechten Herzens," translated in "Werner Forssmann and the Catheterization of the Heart," trans. by John A. Meyer, M.D., *Annals of Thoracic Surgery,* vol. 49, 1990, p. 497

10. Forssmann, *Experiments on Myself,* p. 83

11. Forssmann, *Experiments on Myself,* p. 83

12. Forssmann, *Experiments on Myself,* p. 84

13. "Doctor Gets Catheter by a Vein to Heart," *New York Times,* Nov. 4, 1929, p. 8

14. Allen B. Weisse M.D., Andre Cournand interview, *Conversations in Medicine* (New York: New York University, 1984), pp. 120–121

15. Lawrence K. Altman M.D. "Daring Experiment Aided Heart Care," *New York Times,* July 10, 1979, p. C3

16. Yale Enson and Mary Dickinson Chamberlin, "Cournand & Richards and the Bellevue Hospital Cardiopulmonary Laboratory," *Columbia Magazine,* Fall 2001

17. Dickinson Richards, Nobel speech.

18. "Janet S. Baldwin, Physician, 50, Dies," *New York Times,* Sept. 19, 1958, p. 28

19. Felix Belair Jr., "3 Win Nobel Prize for Heart Study," *New York Times,* Oct. 19, 1956, p. 1

Never Say Die

1. "Aim Is Barnyard, Not Nursery," *The New York Times,* Mar. 3, 1997, p. B6

2. S.M. Silladsen, "Nuclear transplantation in sheep embryos," *Nature,* vol 320, Mar. 6, 1986, pp. 63–64

3. Gina Kolata, *The Road to Dolly,* (New York: William Morrow, 1998), p. 187

4. "Aim Is Barnyard, Not Nursery," p. B6

5. Martin Fransman, "Designing Dolly: interactions between economics, technology, and science and the evolution of hybrid institutions," *Research Policy* vol. 30, 2001, pp. 264–66

6. Robert Lee Hotz, "Caught in a Furor of His Own Creation," *The Los Angeles Times* Mar. 6, 1997, p. 1.

7. "Scientists, Copying Cells, Produce Identical Sheep," *The New York Times,* Mar. 7, 1996, B14.

8. I. Wilmut, A. E. Schnieke, J. McWhir, A .J. Kind, K. H. S. Campbell, "Viable offspring derived from fetal and adult mammalian cells," *Nature,* vol. 385, Feb. 27, 1997, p. 812

9. Robin McKie, "Goodbye Dolly," London *Observer,* Feb. 16, 2003, p. 28

Endnotes

10. James Meek, "Tears of a Clone," *Manchester Guardian,* April 19, 2002, p. II–2
11. Gina Kolata, "Scientist Reports First Cloning Ever of Adult Mammal," *The New York Times,* Feb. 23, 1997, p. 22
12. Bruce Wallace, "The Dolly Debate," *Maclean's* vol. 110, Mar. 10, 1997, p. 55.
13. Harold T. Shapiro, "Ethical and Policy Issues of Human Cloning," *Science,* vol. 277, July 11, 1997, p. 195
14. Robert Langreth, "Science: Mice Are Cloned, Indicating Dolly Wasn't a Fluke," *Wall Street Journal,* July 23, 1998, p. B1.
15. Tim Radford, "Scientist of 'Dolly the Sheep' fame asked by families to clone their close relatives," *Manchester Guardian,* June 26, 1997, p. 1
16. "A Quiet Scientist in the Public Eye," *The New York Times,* Mar. 3, 1998, p. B7
17. Hotz, "Caught in a Furor of His Own Creation," p. 1
18. Ian Wilmut, "Dolly's creator on the ethics of cloning," *American Enterprise,* vol. 9, no 5, Sept/Oct, 1998, p. 57
19. "Don't Clone People, says man who made Dolly," *Times* (London), Mar. 29, 2001, p. 10
20. Wilmut, "Dolly's creator on the ethics of cloning," p. 58
21. Meek, "Tears of a Clone," p. II–2

II. Germ Theory

Perfect Focus

1. Arthur K. Wheelock Jr., *Vermeer,* (New York: Harry Abrams, 1981), pp. 136–8
2. J. van Zuylen, "The Microscopes of Antony van Leeuwenhoek," *Journal of Microscopy,* vol 121, pt. 3, March 1981, p. 309
3. Elmer Bendiner, "The Man Who Did Not Invent the Microscope," *Hospital Practice,* August 1984, p. 168
4. Elmer Bendiner, "The Man Who Did Not Invent the Microscope," *Hospital Practice,* August 1984, p. 165
5. Dr. John Bethune Stein, "On the Trail of Van Leeuwenhoek," *Scientific Monthly* vol. 32, no. 2 Feb. 1931, p. 11
6. Brian J. Ford, *Single Lens* (New York: Harper & Row, 1985), p. 19
7. Gustave Fassin, "Something about the Early Microscope," *Scientific Monthly,* vol. 38, no. 5, May, 1934, p. 457
8. Bendiner, "The Man Who Did Not Invent the Microscope," p. 174
9. Reginald S. Clay and Thomas H. Court, *The History of the Microscope* (London: Charles Griffin & Co., 1932), p. 26
10. Ford, *Single Lens,* p. 4
11. Dr. John Bethune Stein, "On the Trail of Van Leeuwenhoek," *Scientific Monthly* vol. 32, no. 2 Feb. 1931, p. 118
12. Leeuwenhoek, Antoni van, *A specimen of some observations made by a microscope* (London : The Society, 1673
13. L. E. Casida Jr., "Leeuwenhoek's Observation of Bacteria," *Science,* vol. 192, no. 4246, Jun 25, 1976, p. 193
14. Stein, "On the Trail of Van Leeuwenhoek," p. 123

15. Edward G. Ruestow, "Images and Ideas: Leeuwenhoek's Perception of the Spermatozoa," *Journal of the History of Biology,* vol 16, no. 2, pp. 191–4

16. L.C. Palm, "Leeuwenhoek and Other Dutch Correspondents of the Royal Society," *Notes and Records of the Royal Society of London,* vol. 43, no. 2 July 1989, p. 193

17. Stein, "On the Trail of Van Leeuwenhoek," p. 122

18. Edward G. Ruestow, "Images and Ideas: Leeuwenhoek's Perception of the Spermatozoa," *Journal of the History of Biology,* vol 16, no. 2, pp. 191–4

19. Palm, "Leeuwenhoek and Other Dutch Correspondents of the Royal Society," p. 196

20. Bendiner, "The Man Who Did Not Invent the Microscope," p. 165

21. Palm, "Leeuwenhoek and Other Dutch Correspondents of the Royal Society," p. 194

22. Clay and Court, *The History of the Microscope,* p. 34

Too Much Trouble

1. Peter Baldry, *Unknown Enemy* (Cambridge: Cambridge Univ., 1965), p. 12

2. J.M. Duncan, *On the Mortality of Childbed and Maternity Hospitals* (New York: William Wood, 1871), quoted in Edwin F. Daily, M.D., "Notes on Puerperal Fever," *Journal of the American Medical Association,* vol. 121, Mar. 27, 1943, p. 1007

3. "CDC releases new hand-hygiene guidelines," press release, Oct. 25, 2002, Centers for Disease Control (Atlanta)

4. Didier Pittet, M.D., MS; Phillippe Mourouga M.D. Msc.; Thomas V. Perneger, M.D,. Ph.D, et al, "Compliance with Handwashing in a Teaching Hospital," *Annals of Internal Medicine,* vol 130, no. 2, Jan 19, 1999.

5. Richard P. Wenzel and Michael B. Edmond, "The Impact of Hospital-Acquired Bloodstream Infections," *Emerging Infectious Diseases,* vol. 7, no. 2, Mar.–Apr., 2001.

6. Pittet, et al.

7. Frank G. Slaughter, M.D., *Immortal Magyar: Semmelweis, Conqueror of Childbed Fever,* (New York: Henry Schuman, 1950), p. 24

8. K. Codell Carter and Barbara R. Carter, *Childbed Fever: A Scientific Biography of Ignaz Semmelweis* (Westport, Conn.: Greenwood, 1994), p. 44

9. E. Robert Wiese, "Semmelweis," *Annals of Medical History,* n.s. II, no. 1, Jan. 1930, p. 84

10. Carter and Carter, *Childbed Fever* p. 27

11. Charles B. Johnson, "A Medical Martyr of the Eighteen Sixties," *Illinois Medical Journal* Feb. 1929, p. 145

12. Johnson, "A Medical Martyr of the Eighteen Sixties," p. 145

13. Ignaz Semmelweis, *The Etiology, Concept and Prophylaxis of Childbed Fever,* K. Codell Carter, editor and trans. (Madison: Univ. Of Wisc., 1983), p. 70

14. Carter and Carter, *Childbed Fever,* p. 29

15. Wiese, "Semmelweis," p. 82

16. Alexander Gordon, *A Treatise on the Epidemic Puerperal Fever of Aberdeen* (1795), pp. 445–500, quoted in Slaughter, p. 36.

17. Oliver Wendell Holmes "The Contagiousness of Puerperal Fever," (1855 version) reprinted in *The Works of Oliver Wendell Holmes,* (Boston: Houghton Mifflin, 1892) vol. 9, p. 163

Endnotes

18. Edwin F. Daily, M.D., "Notes on Puerperal Fever, 1843–1943," *Journal of the American Medical Association,* vol. 121, Mar. 27, 1943, p. 1006
19. Wiese, "Semmelweis," p. 82
20. Ignác Fülöp Semmelweis, Frank P. Murphy, M.D., trans., *The Etiology, the Concept and the Prophylaxis of Childbed Fever* (Birmingham: Classic of Medicine Library, 1981), p. 356
21. Semmelweis, *The Etiology, the Concept and the Prophylaxis of Childbed Fever,* p. 376
22. Carter and Carter, *Childbed Fever,* p. 33
23. Carter and Carter, *Childbed Fever,* p. 51
24 Johnson, "A Medical Martyr of the Eighteen Sixties," p. 146
25. Daily, "Notes on Puerperal Fever, 1843–1943," p. 1006
26. Carter and Carter, *Childbed Fever,* p. 69
27. Sherwin B. Nuland, M.D., "The Enigma of Semmelweis — an Interpretation," preface in Ignác Fülöp Semmelweis, *The Etiology, the Concept and the Prophylaxis of Childbed Fever* (Birmingham: Classic of Medicine Library, 1981), p. xl
28. Daily, "Notes on Puerperal Fever, 1843–1943," p. 1007

Public Enemy

1. Ragnhild Münch, "Robert Koch," *Microbes and Infections,* vol. 5, 2003, p. 72
2. Thomas M. Daniel, *Captain Death: The Story of Tuberculosis* (Rochester, N.Y.: University of Rochester, 1997 p. 74
3. "The Bacteriologist Who Revolutionized Medicine," *Current Literature,* vol. 49, no.1, July, 1910, p. 56
4. Robert Koch, *The Aetiology of Tuberculosis: a translation from the German of the original paper announcing the discovery of Tubercle Bacillus,* trans. By Dr. and Mrs. Max Pinner (New York: National Tuberculosis Assoc., 1932), p. 23
5. Koch, *The Aetiology of Tuberculosis,* p. 46
6. Münch, "Robert Koch," p. 72
7. Münch, "Robert Koch," p. 72–3
8. Herbert A. Lechevalier and Morris Solotorovsky, *Three Centuries of Microbiology,* (New York: McGraw-Hill, 1965), p. 63
9. Thomas M. Daniel, *Captain Death: The Story of Tuberculosis* (Rochester, N.Y.: University of Rochester, 1997
10. Lechevalier and Morris, *Three Centuries of Microbiology,* p. 69
11. Dr. Robert Koch, "Investigations in the Etiology of Traumatic Infective Diseases, trans. By W. Watson Cheyne (Birmingham: Classics of Medicine Library, 1991), p. 21
12. Jay Arthur Myers, *Fighters of Fate,* (Freeport, N.Y.: Books for Libraries, 1969)
13. Thomas Dormandy, *White Death: A History of Tuberculosis* (New York: New York University, 1999), p. xiii
14. Koch, *The Aetiology of Tuberculosis,* p. 47
15. "Koch and his Modified Snake-bite," *Review of Reviews,* vol. 3, no. 16, April 1891, p. 369
16. Arthur Conan Doyle, "Dr. Koch and His Cure," *Review of Reviews,* vol. 2, no. 12, Dec. 1890, p. 555
17. Lechevalier and Morris, *Three Centuries of Microbiology,* p. 110

Trailing Death

1. Lee K. Frankel, Ph.D., "Science and the Public Health," *American Journal of Public Health,* vol. 5, no. 4, April 1915, p. 289

2. Douglas Farah, "Patients Laud Cuban AIDS Care," *Washington Post,* Aug. 11, 1993, p. 1

3. Tim Golden, "Patients Pay High price in Cuba's War on AIDS," *New York Times,* Oct. 16, 1995, p. A10

4. Julia Preston, "Cuba's Push to Isolate AIDS," *Washington Post,* Feb. 14, 1989, p. WH6

5. *Lincoln Library of Essential Information* (Buffalo: Frontier Press, 1928), p. 2092

6. "Ithaca's Typhoid Epidemic," *New York Times,* Mar. 3, 1903, p. 1; "Attendance at Cornell," *ibid,* Apr. 15, 1903, p. 8

7. "Ithaca as an Object Lesson," *New York Times,* Apr. 27, 1903, p. 6

8. " 'Typhoid Mary' has Reappeared," *New York Times Sunday Magazine,* April 4, 1915, p. 3

9. "Mary Mallon," *American Journal of Public Health,* vol. 29, Jan. 1939, p. 67

10. William H. Park, M.D., "Typhoid Bacilli Carriers," *Journal of the American Medical Association,* vol. 51, no. 12, September 19, 1908, p.981

11. Major George A. Soper, "Typhoid Mary," *Military Surgeon,* vol. XLV, no. 1, July 1919

12. " 'Typhoid Mary' has Reappeared," *New York Times Sunday Magazine,* April 4, 1915, p. 3

13. Major George A. Soper, "Typhoid Mary," *Military Surgeon,* vol. XLV, no. 1, July 1919

14. Major Soper, ibid.

15. Major Soper, ibid.

16. William H. Park, M.D., "Typhoid Bacilli Carriers," *Journal of the American Medical Association,* vol. 51, no. 12, September 19, 1908, p.981

17. Park, ibid.

18. Letter to the Editor, signed "A New Thought Student," *New York Times,* July 2, 1909, p. 6

19. " 'Typhoid Mary' Must Stay," *New York Times,* July 17, 1909, p. 3

20. "Guide a Walking Typhoid Factory," *New York Times,* Dec. 2, 1910, p. 6

21. " 'Typhoid Mary' Freed," *New York Times,* Feb. 21, 1910, p. 18

22. "A Pressing Problem," *American Journal of Public Health,* vol. 5, no 4, Apr. 1915, p. 313

23. "Hospital Epidemic from Typhoid Mary," *New York Times,* Mar. 28, 1915, p. 11

24. Major George A. Soper, "Typhoid Mary," *Military Surgeon,* vol. XLV, no. 1, July 1919

25. "Mary Mallon," *American Journal of Public Health,* vol. 29, Jan. 1939, p. 66

26. "Mary Mallon," *American Journal of Public Health,* vol. 29, Jan. 1939, p. 67

Magic Bullets

Worldly Wise

1. Robert Halsband, *The Life of Lady Mary Wortley Montagu* (Oxford: Clarendon Press, 1956), p. 75

2. Lady Mary Wortley Montagu, letter to Alexander Pope, June 17, 1717, *The*

Endnotes

Complete Letters of Lady Mary Wortley Montagu, vol. I, edited by Robert Halsband (Oxford: Clarendon Press, 1965), pp. 365–6

3. Halsband, *The Life of Lady Mary Wortley Montagu,* p. 70

4. Thomas B. Macaulay, *The History of England from the Accession of James II,* (New York: E.P. Dutton, 1910)

5. "Smallpox overview," Centers for Disease Control, U.S. Department of Health and Human Services, Dec. 9, 2002

6. Nicolau Barquet, M.D., and Pere Domingo, M.D., "Smallpox: The Triumph over the Most Terrible of the Ministers of Death," *Annals of Internal Medicine* vol. 127 Oct. 15, 1997, p. 636

7. Halsband, *The Life of Lady Mary Wortley Montagu,* p. 53

8. Genevieve Miller, "Putting Lady Mary in Her Place: A Discussion of Historical Causation," *Bulletin of the History of Medicine,* vol 55, 1981, p. 4

9. Lady Mary Montagu, letter to [Sarah Chiswell], April 1 [1717], Robert Halsband, editor, *The Complete Letters of Lady Mary Wortley Montagu* (Oxford: Clarendon Press, 1965), pp. 338–9

10. Lady Mary Montagu, letter to [Sarah Chiswell], April 1 [1717], ibid

11. Halsband, *The Life of Lady Mary Wortley Montagu,* p. 80

12. Lady Mary Montagu, letter to Edward Wortley Montagu, Mar. 23 [1718], Robert Halsband, editor, *The Complete Letters of Lady Mary Wortley Montagu* (Oxford: Clarendon Press, 1965), pp. 392

13. Barquet and Domingo, "Smallpox: The Triumph over the Most Terrible of the Ministers of Death," p. 637

14. Guy Williams, "The Age of Agony," (Chicago: Academy Press, 1986), p.73

15. Isobel Grundy, "Montagu's Variolation," *Endeavor,* vol. 24, no. 1, Mar. 2000, p. 4

Tag Ook

1. "Brings From Europe Ehrlich's Remedy," *New York Times,*, Oct. 5, 1910, p. 5

2. Frederick H. Baker, M.D. "Control of Venereal Diseases by Health Departments," *American Journal of Public Health,* Apr. 1915, vol. 5, no. 4, p. 290–1

3. Allan M. Brandt, "The Syphilis Epidemic and its Relation to AIDS," *Science,* vol. 239, Jan. 22, 1988, p. 376

4. Baker, M.D. "Control of Venereal Diseases by Health Departments," p. 293

5. Dr. Thomas Parran, "Syphilis: A Public Health Problem," *Science,* vol. 87, no. 2251, Feb. 18, 1939, p. 147

6. Mark Rose, "Origins of Syphilis," *Archeology,* vol. 50, no. 1, Feb. 1997

7. Brandt, "The Syphilis Epidemic and its Relation to AIDS," p. 239

8. Margaret Goldsmith, "Paul Ehrlich," *Twelve Jews,* edited by Hector Bolitho (Freeport, N.Y.: Books for Libraries Press, 1967, orig. pub. 1934), p. 78

9. Martha Marquardt, *Paul Ehrlich* (London: William Heinemann, 1949), p. 15

10. Marquardt, *Paul Ehrlich,* p. 4–5

11. Goldsmith, "Paul Ehrlich," *Twelve Jews,* p. 66

12. Carl Ludwig Schleich, *Those Were Good Days!* Trans. By Bernard Miall, (New York: Norton, 1936), p. 233

13. Fritz Stern, *Einstein's German World* (Princeton, N.J.: Princeton University, 1999), p. 22

14. Marquardt, *Paul Ehrlich,* p. 119

15. "606 As Malaria Cure," *New York Times,*, Oct. 3, 1910, p. 4

16. "Edison Sees 1912 Great, Minus Greed," *New York Times,* Jan. 3, 1912, p. 6

17. "World Doctors Hail Ehrlich As Hero," *New York Times,*, Aug. 9, 1913, p. 10

18. Stern, *Einstein's German World,* p. 28

19. Schleich, *Those Were Good Days!* p. 236

Et Al

1. Selman A. Waksman, *My Life With the Microbes* (New York: Simon & Schuster), 1954, p. 25

2. "Immigration to United States for Selected Years," *Lincoln Library of Essential Information* (Buffalo: Frontier Press, 1928), p. 2100

3. Waksman, *My Life With the Microbes,* p. 68

4. Selman A. Waksman, "What Is Humus?" *Proceedings of the National Academy of Sciences of the U.S.A,* vol. 11, no. 8, Aug. 15, 1925, pp. 463–468

5. Selman A. Waksman, "Soil Microbiology as a Field of Science," *Science,* vol. 102, no. 2649, Oct. 5, 1945, p. 339–344

6. Waksman, "Soil Microbiology as a Field of Science," p. 339

7. Selman A. Waksman, "The Soil Population," *Proceedings of the National Academy of Sciences of the U.S.A,* vol. 11, no. 8, Aug. 15, 1925, pp. 476–481

8. Harry Gilroy, "Waksman and 10,000 Microbes," *New York Times Magazine,* Nov. 2, 1950, p. 20

9. Doris Jones, lecture notes quoted in Frank Ryan, M.D., *The Forgotten Plague* (Boston: Little Brown, 1992), pp. 212–3

10. Selman A. Waksman, *The Conquest of Tuberculosis* (Berkeley: Univ. Of Calif., 1964), p. 113

11. Eileen Gregory, interview *Mavericks, Miracles, and Medicine* television documentary manuscript, p. 31

12. Veronique Mistiaen, "Time, and the great healer," *Manchester Guardian,* November 2, 2002

13. Doris Jones, H. J. Metzger, Albert Schatz, Selman Waksman, "Control of Gram-Negative Bacteria in Experimental Animals by Streptomycin," *Science,* vol. 100, no 2588, Aug. 4, 1944, p. 103–105

14. Schatz, A.; Bugie, E.,; Waksman, S.A., "Streptomycin, a substance exhibiting antibiotic activity against gram-positive and gram-negative bacteria," *Proceedings for Experimental Biology and Medicine,* vol. 55, 1944, pp. 66–9

15. H. Corwin and William H. Feldman, "Observations on Chemotherapy of Clinical & Experimental Tuberculosis," Mayo Clinic *Proceedings,* July, 1945, pp. 918–22

16. "Streptomycin Looks Better," *Time,* vol. 46, Oct. 15, 1945, p. 94

17. WHO Table (1962), reprinted in Waksman, *The Conquest of Tuberculosis,* p. 135

18. Mistiaen, "Time, and the great healer"

19. "Streptomycin Pays," *Time,* vol. 53, May 16, 1949, p. 87

20. *Albert Schatz vs Selman A. Waksman and Rutgers Research and Endowment Foundation* Rutgers University Archives and Special Collections.

Endnotes

21. "Strepto-settlement," *Time,* vol. 57, Jan. 8, 1951, p. 32
22. "Streptomycin Suit Is Labeled 'Baseless,' " *New York Times,* Mar. 13, 1950, p. 31
23. Waksman, *The Conquest of Tuberculosis,* p. 117
24. See notes 12 and 13; also "Selman A. Waksman, H. Christine Reilly, Albert Schatz, "Strain Specificity and Production of Antibiotic Substances, V, Strain Resistance of Bacteria to Antibiotic Substances, Especially to Streptomycin," *Proceedings of the National Academy of Sciences of the United States of America,* vol. 31, no. 6, June 15, 1945, pp. 157–64 and Albert Schatz, Selman A. Waksman, "Strain Specificity and Production of Antibiotic Substances, IV, Variations Among Actinomycetes, with Special Reference to Actinomyces Griseus," *Proceedings of the National Academy of Sciences of the United States of America,* vol. 31, no. 5, May 15, 1945, pp. 129–37
25. Selman A. Waksman, "Microbiology Takes the Stage," *Scientific Monthly,* vol. 79, no. 6, Dec. 1954, p. 358

Battery Operated

1. Lawrence K. Altman, "Heart Pacemakers Stir Medical Revolution," *New York Times,* July 22, 1973, p. 24
2. H.J. Th. Thalen, M.D.;, Jw. vanden Berg, D.Sc; J.N. Homan vander Heide, M.D., J. Nieveen, M.D.; *The Artificial Cardiac Pacemaker* (Baltimore: Charles C. Thomas, 1969), p. 20
3. Thalen et al., *Artificial Cardiac Pacemaker,* p. 33–34
4. Paul M. Zoll, M.D., "Historical Development of Cardiac Pacemakers," *Progress in Cardiovascular Diseases,* vol. 14, no. 5, March 1972, 422
5. Paul Zoll, M.D., "Development of Electric Control of Cardiac Rhythm," *Journal of the American Medical Association* vol. 226, no. 8, Nov. 19, 1973, p. 882
6. Marcel Tuchman, interview, 2002, for television documentary, *Mavericks, Miracles and Medicine,* original transcript
7. Åke Senning, M.D., "Cardiac Pacing in Retrospect," *American Journal of Surgery,* vol. 145, June 1983, p. 735
8. Kim Gamel, "Novel Pacemaker Patient Dead at 86," Associated Press, Jan. 16, 2002
9.. Else-Marie Larsson, interview, 2002, for television documentary, *Mavericks, Miracles, and Medicine,* original transcript, p. 35
10. Senning, "Cardiac Pacing in Retrospect," p. 733
11. Åke Senning, M.D., "Developments in Cardiac Surgery in Stockholm During the Mid and Late 1950's," *Journal of Thoracic and Cardiovascular Surgery,* vol. 98, no. 5, part 2, November 1989, p. 830
12. Senning, "Cardiac Pacing in Retrospect," p. 733
13. Kirk Jeffrey, *Machines in our Hearts* (Baltimore: Johns Hopkins, 2001), p. 90
14. Lars Ryden, Hans Schuller, Berit Larsson, "Arne Larsson," *North American Society of Pacing and Electrophysiology,* website entry.
15. Senning, "Cardiac Pacing in Retrospect," p. 735
16. Else-Marie Larsson, interview, 2002, for television documentary, *Mavericks, Miracles, and Medicine,* original transcript, p. 36

17. Dr. Rune Elmqvist, "Review of Early Pacemaker Development," PACE, vol. 1, Oct.–Dec., 1978, p. 536
18. Lawrence K. Altman, "Paul M. Zoll Is Dead at 87," *New York Times,* Jan 8, 1999, B11
19. Gamel, "Novel Pacemaker Patient Dead at 86" Associated Press, Jan. 16, 2002
20. Lawrence K. Altman, "Heart Pacemakers Stir Medical Revolution," *New York Times,* July 22, 1973, p. 24

IV. The Mind

Organized Brain
1. Sir Charles Symonds, "Thomas Willis, F.R.S.," *Notes and Records of the Royal Society of London,* vol. 15, July, 1960, p. 91
2. Hansruedi Isler, *Thomas Willis, 1621–1675, Doctor and Scientist* (New York: Hofner, 1968), p. 4
3. Kenneth Dewhurst, "Some Letters of Dr. Thomas Willis," *Medical History,* vol. 16, Jan 1972, p. 77
4. Isler, *Thomas Willis, 1621–1675, Doctor and Scientist,* p. 6
5. Isler, *Thomas Willis, 1621–1675, Doctor and Scientist,* p. 18
6. Anthony Wood, *Athenae Oxoniensis: An Exact History of All the Writers and Bishops Who had their Education in the University at Oxford,* quoted in: Sir Charles Symonds, "Thomas Willis, F.R.S.," *Notes and Records of the Royal Society of London,* vol. 15, July, 1960, p. 96
7. 8. Symonds, "Thomas Willis, F.R.S.," p. 92
9. James P.B. O'Connor, "Thomas Willis and the background to *Cerebri Anatome,*" *Journal of the Royal Society of Medicine* vol. 96, Mar. 2003, p. 140
10. William F. Bynum, "The Anatomical Method, Natural Theology, and the Functions of the Brain," *Isis,* vol. 64, no. 4, Dec., 1973, p. 447
11. O'Connor, "Thomas Willis and the background to *Cerebri Anatome,*" p. 141
12. Devera G. Schoenberg M.S., and Bruce S. Schoenberg, M.D., "The Death of the Birth of Neurology," *Surgical Neurology* vol. 4, Oct., 1975, p. 405
13. Isler, *Thomas Willis, 1621–1675,* p. 104
14. Bynum, "The Anatomical Method, Natural Theology, and the Functions of the Brain," p. 459
15. O'Connor, "Thomas Willis and the background to *Cerebri Anatome,*" p. 142
16. M. J. Eadie, "A pathology of the animal spirits—the clinical neurology of Thomas Willis" Part I., *Journal of Clinical Neuroscience,* vol. 10, 2003, pp. 17–21
17. Symonds, "Thomas Willis, F.R.S.," p. 95
18. Bynum, "The Anatomical Method, Natural Theology, and the Functions of the Brain," p. 447

Lost in Thought
1. Peter McCandless, "Mesmerism and Phrenology in antebellum Charleston," *Journal of Southern History,* vol 58, no. 2, May, 1992, p. 209
2. Paul Thompson, Tyrone D. Cannon and Arthur W. Toga, Mapping genetic

Endnotes

influences on human brain structure," *Annals of Medicine*, 2002, vol. 34, pp. 523–4

3. Samuel H. Greenblatt M.D., "Phrenology in the Science and Culture of the 19th Century," *Neurosurgery*, vol. 37, no. 4, Oct., 1995, p. 791

4. Owsei Temkin, "Gall and the Phrenological Movement," *Bulletin of the History of Medicine*, vol. 21, no. 3, May–June, 1947, p. 279

5. S. Zola-Morgan, "Localization of Brain Function: The Legacy of Franz Joseph Gall (1758–1828)," *Annual Review of Neuroscience*, vol. 18, 1995, p. 362

6. Martin Straum, "Physiognomy and Phrenology at the Paris Athénée," *Journal of the History of Ideas*, vol 56, no 3, Jul, 1995, p. 447

7. Angus McLaren, "A Prehistory of the Social Sciences," *Comparative Studies in Society and History*, vol. 23, no. 1, Jan. 1981, p. 5

8. Zola-Morgan, "Localization of Brain Function," p. 364

9. Greenblatt M.D., "Phrenology in the Science and Culture of the 19th Century," p. 792

10. Straum, "Physiognomy and Phrenology at the Paris Athénée," p. 450

11. Zola-Morgan, "Localization of Brain Function," p. 363

12. Straum, "Physiognomy and Phrenology at the Paris Athénée," p. 447

13. Zola-Morgan, "Localization of Brain Function," p. 373

14. McCandless, "Mesmerism and Phrenology in antebellum Charleston," p. 199

15. Fred G. Barker, M.D., "Phineas among the phrenologists: the American crowbar case and nineteenth-century theories of cerebral localization," *Journal of Neurosurgery*, vol. 82, April, 1995, p. 674

Ether Frolic

1. Jack Rohan, *Yankee Arms Maker* (New York: Harper & Bros., 1935), p. 26–50

2. Humphry Davy, "Researches on Nitrous-Oxide Gas," *Proceedings of the Royal Society*, 1799, p. 566

3. "Ether and Chloroform," *Dublin Review*, Sept. 1850, p. 235

4. E. H. Poole and F. J. McGowan, *Surgery at the New York Hospital One Hundred Years Ago* (New York: Paul Hoeber, 1929), p. 1–2.

5. John H. Ashhurst Jr., M.D., "Surgery Before the Days of Anesthesia," *The Semi-Centennial of Anesthesia* (Massachusetts General Hospital, 1896), pp. 31–2

6. Crawford W. Long, "An Account of the First Use of Sulphuric Ether," *Southern Medical and Surgical Journal 5* (1849), reprinted in The History of Anesthesiology reprint series no. 1 (Oak Ridge, Ill.: Wood Library-Museum, 1992), pp. 3–13

7. Gardner Q. Colton, "The Invention of Anesthesia," letter to the editor, the *New York Times*, Feb. 5, 1862.

8. Reginald Fitz, "The Value of Imponderables," *New England Journal of Medicine*, 236, no. 16 (Apr. 1947), p. 557

9. Daniel D. Slade, "The First Capital Operation Under the Influence of Ether," *Scribner's Magazine* July 1892, p. 521

10. Oliver Wendell Holmes to William T. G. Morton, reprinted in Albert H. Miller, M.D., "The Origin of the Word, 'Anesthesia,'" *Boston Medical and Surgical Journal*, 197, no. 26 (Dec. 1927), p. 122

11. "Distressing Case of a Suicide," *New York Tribune,* Jan. 25, 1848, p. 2; also, *New York Herald,* Jan. 25, 1848, p. 2
12. "The Death of Professor Morton," *New York Herald,* July 17, 1868, p. 5; also "Death of Prof. Morton," *New York Times,* July 17, 1868, p. 5, also, "Sudden Death of Dr. Morton," *Boston Transcript,* July 17, 1868, p. 2
13. Ellen Tucker Emerson, *The Life of Lidian Jackson Emerson,* edited by Delores Bird Carpenter (Boston: Twayne, 1980), pp. 310–11.

Human Feeling

1. Kenneth L. Tyler M.D. and Rolf Malessa, M.D., "The Goltz-Ferrier debates and the triumph of cerebral localizationalist theory," *Neurology,* vol. 55, Oct. 2000, p. 1017. Most of the factual description of the debate is drawn from this article.
2. Ronald S. Fishman, "Brain Wars: Passion and conflict in the localization of vision in the brain," *Documenta Opthalmologica,* vol. 89, 1995, p. 175
3. "Sir David Ferrier," *The New York Times,* Mar. 20, 1928, p. 22.
4. Robert M. Young, "The Functions of the Brain, Gall to Ferrier (1808–1886)," *Isis,* vol. 59, no. 3, Autumn, 1968, p. 263
5. Henry G. Heffner, Ph.D., "Ferrier and the Study of Auditory Cortex," *Archives of Neurology,* vol. 44, Feb, 1987, p. 219
6. Richard D. French, *Antivivisection and Medical Science in Victorian Society* (Princeton: Princeton U., 1975), p. 200
7. French, *Antivivisection and Medical Science in Victorian Society,* p. 281
8. Moira Ferguson, *Animal Advocacy and Englishwomen* (Ann Arbor: Univ. Of Michigan, 1998), p. 112.
9. Stephen Coleridge, *Vivisection: A Heartless Science* (London: John Lane, 1916), p. 64
10. George Huggan, letter to the London *Morning Post,* Feb. 2, 1875, reprinted in: Albert Leffingwell, *An Ethical Problem: Sidelights Upon Scientific Experimentation on Man and Animals* (London: G. Bell, 1914), p. 94
11. F. Barbara Orlans, *In the Name of Science: Issues in Responsible Animal Experimentation* (New York: Oxford, 1993), p. 8
12. Leffingwell, *An Ethical Problem,* p. 97
13. Leffingwell, *An Ethical Problem,* p. 95
14. French, *Antivivisection and Medical Science in Victorian Society,* p. 120
15. Mary T. Phillips and Jeri Sechzer, *Animal Research and Ethical Conflict* (New York: Springer-Verlag, 1989), p. 9
16. French, *Antivivisection and Medical Science in Victorian Society,* p. 195
17. Coleridge, *Vivisection: A Heartless Science,* p. 65
18. Ferguson, *Animal Advocacy and Englishwomen,* p. 114
19. Ferguson, *Animal Advocacy and Englishwomen,* p. 113
20. "The Charge Against Professor Ferrier," *The Times* (London), Nov. 18, 1881, p. 10
21. Frederic Rowland Marvin, letter, April 6, 1904, *The New York Times,* April 16, 1904, p. BR266
22. Fishman, "Brain Wars: Passion and conflict in the localization of vision in the brain," p. 183

Endnotes

23. Douglas B. Kirkpatrick, M.D., "The First Primary Brain-Tumor Operation," *Journal of Neurosurgery,* vol. 61, 1984, p. 810

V. Toward Better Surgery
Transfusion of Murder
1. Hebbel E. Hoff, "Jean-Baptiste Denis," *Dictionary of Scientific Biography,* vol. 4, p. 37
2. N.S.R. Maluf, "History of Blood Transfusion," *Journal of the History of Medicine,* Jan. 1954, p. 60
3. Maluf, "History of Blood Transfusion," p. 63
4. Anita Guerrini, "The Ethics of Animal Experimentation in Seventeenth-Century England," *Journal of the History of Ideas,* vol. 50, no. 3, Jul–Sep, 1989, p 403
5. A.D. Farr, "The First Human Blood Transfusion," *Medical History,* vol. 24, 1980, p. 160; translation was corrected to reflect standard spelling
6. Farr, "The First Human Blood Transfusion," p. 144
7. M. Whitten, M.D., J. Patrick M.D. "The Origins of Blood Transfusion: Early History," *American Surgeon,* vol. 68, no. 1, p. 99
8. Wise and O'Leary, "The Origins of Blood Transfusion," p. 99
9. Maluf, "History of Blood Transfusion," p. 67
10. Corinne S. Wood, "A Short History of Blood Transfusion," *Transfusion,* vol. 7, July–Aug. 1967, p. 300

Master of the System
1. "Lemon juice 'cuts the risk of DVT' " *The Times* (London) August 20, 2001
2. "Flight with a Silent Killer," Coventry (UK) *Evening Telegraph,* Dec. 2, 2002
3. Jane Brody, "On the Long Flights, Take Steps, Lots of Them," *New York Times,* Dec. 17, 2002, p. F8
4. A. Dickson Wright, foreword; Kenneth J. Franklin, *William Harvey, Englishman,* (London: MacGibbon & Kee, 1961), p. 9
5. Louis Chauvois, *William Harvey: His Life and Times* (New York: Philosophical Library, 1957; translated from the French), p. 39
6. Chauvois, p. 44
7. D.W. Thompson, translator, *The Works of Aristotle,* vol. IV (London: Oxford University Press, 1910)
8. Mark Graubard, *Circulation and Respiration: Evolution of an Idea* (New York: Harcourt, Brace and World, 1964), p. 82
9. Chauvois, p. 67
10. Robert Boyle, 1688, reprinted in Kenneth Franklin, *William Harvey, Englishman* (London: MacGibbon & Kee, 1961), pp. 51–2
11. Gweneth Whittridge, *William Harvey and the Circulation of the Blood,* (New York: American Elsevier, 1971), p. 111
12. Charles Webster, "William Harvey and the Crisis of Medicine in Jacobean England,", Jerome J. Bylebyl, editor, *William Harvey and His Age,* (Baltimore: Johns Hopkins Univ., 1979), pp. 1–16

13. Geoffrey Keynes, *The Personality of William Harvey,* (Cambridge: Cambridge University, 1949), pp. 13–14

14. Kenneth D. Keele, *William Harvey: the Man, the Physician, and the Scientist* (New York: Nelson, 1965), p. 88

15. Archibald Malloch, *William Harvey,* (New York: Paul B. Hoebler, 1929), p. 13.

16. Eric Neil, *William Harvey and the Circulation of the Blood,* (London: Picory Press, 1975), p. 44

17. William Harvey, *De Motu cordis,* preface, translation in Gweneth Whittridge, *William Harvey and the Circulation of the Blood,* (New York: American Elsevier, 1971), p. 104

18. William Harvey, *De Motu Cordis,* trans. By Robert Willis, reprinted in Robert Maynard Hutchins, Editor-in-chief, *Great Books of the Western World,* (Chicago: William Benton, 1952), vol.28, p. 274.

19. Kenneth J. Franklin, *William Harvey, Englishman* (London: MacGibbon & Kee, 1961), p. 70.

20. John Aubrey on William Harvey, reprinted in Keynes, *Life of William Harvey,* appendix I, p. 435.

21. William J. Ford, "Old Parr," *Bulletin of the History of Machine,* vol. 24, no. I, Jan–Feb, 1950, pp. 219–226.

Long Way to Bypass

1. John H. Gibbon, Jr., "The Development of the Heart-Lung Apparatus," *Review of Surgery,* July–August, 1970, p. 232

2. Harris B. Shumacker, Jr. M.D., *A Dream of the Heart, The Life of John H. Gibbon Jr.* (Santa Barbara: Fithian Press, 1999), p. 80

3. John H. Gibbon Jr., "The Development of the Heart-Lung Apparatus," *American Journal of Surgery* vol 135, May 1973, p. 609

4. John H. Gibbon, Jr., "Application of a Mechanical Heart and Lung Apparatus to Cardiac Surgery," *Minnesota Medicine,* vol. 37, no. 3, Mar. 1954, p. 171

5. John H. Gibbon Jr. "The Maintenance of Life During Experimental Occlusion of the Pulmonary Artery Followed by Survival," *Surgery, Gynecology & Obstetrics* vol. 69, no. 5, Nov, 1939, p. 602

6. John H. Gibbon Jr., "The Development of the Heart-Lung Apparatus," *American Journal of Surgery* vol 135, May 1973, p. 616

7. John H. Gibbon, Jr., "The Development of the Heart-Lung Apparatus," *Review of Surgery,* July–August, 1970, p. 236

8. John H. Gibbon, Jr., "The Development of the Heart-Lung Apparatus," *Review of Surgery,* July–August, 1970, p. 238

9. John H. Gibbon, Jr., "The Development of the Heart-Lung Apparatus," *Review of Surgery,* July–August, 1970, p. 239

10. John H. Gibbon, Jr., "The Development of the Heart-Lung Apparatus," *Review of Surgery,* July–August, 1970, p. 239

11. Harris B. Shumacker, Jr. M.D., *A Dream of the Heart, The Life of John H. Gibbon Jr.* (Santa Barbara: Fithian Press, 1999), p. 278–9

Endnotes

12. Richard Bing M.D., "John H. Gibbon Jr.: Cardiopulmonary Bypass — Triumph of Perseverence and Character," *Clinical Cardiology* vol. 17, 1994, p. 457

A Bit of Life

1. John P. Merrill, M.D.; Joseph E. Murray, M.D.; and J. Hartwell Harrison, M.D., "Successful Homotransplantation of the Human Kidney Between Identical Twins," *Journal of the American Medical Association,* vol. 160, no. 4, Jan. 28, 1956, pp. 277–8
2. Roy Yorke Calne, *Renal Transplantation,* (London: Edward Arnold, 1967), p. 4
3. David Hamilton, "Kidney Transplantation: A History," in *Kidney Transplantation: Principle and Practice,* edited by Peter J. Morris, Ph.D. (Phila: W. B. Saunders, 1994), p. 4
4. Lawrence K. Altman, "Dr. John Merrill, Transplant Pioneer, Dies in Boating Mishap," the *New York Times,* April 10, 1984, p. B10
5. Jean Hamburger, M.D.; Jean Crosnier, M.D.; Jean Dormont, M.D., Jean-François Bach, M.D.; *Renal Transplantation, Theory and Practice* (Baltimore: Williams and Wilkins, 1972), p. vi
6. Joseph E. Murray, M.D.; John P. Merrill, M.D.; and J. Hartwell Harrison, M.D., "Renal Homotransplantation in Identical Twins," *Surgical Forum,* vol. 6, 1955, p. 432
7. Joseph E. Murray, M.D.; John P. Merrill, M.D.; and J. Hartwell Harrison, M.D., "Renal Transplantation Between Seven Pairs of Identical Twins," *Annals of Surgery,* vol. 148, no. 3, Sept. 1958, p. 346
8. Dr. Joseph Murray, *Surgery for the Soul, Reflections on a Curious Career,* (Boston: Boston Medical Library, 2001), p. 75
9. Ronald Herrick, interview with Documania Films, interview transcript, p. 6
10. Murray, Merrill, Harrison, "Renal Homotransplantation in Identical Twins," p. 433
11. Murray, *Surgery for the Soul,* p.77
12. Ronald Herrick, interview with Documania Films, episode script, p. 26
13. Murray, *Surgery for the Soul,* p. 86
14. Murray, Merrill, Harrison, "Renal Homotransplantation in Identical Twins," p. 434
15. Robert K. Plumb, "Man's Life Saved by Twin's Kidney," *New York Times,* Nov. 3, 1955, p. 33
16. Ron Shapiro, M.D.; Richard Simmons, M.D.; and Thomas E. Starzl, M.D., *Renal Transplantation,* (Stamford, Conn. Appelton & Lange, 1997), pp. 30–31; also Joseph E. Murray, M.D.; Nicholas L. Tilney, M.D.; and Richard E. Wilson, M.D., *Annals of Surgery.* Vol 184, no. 5, Nov. 1976, pp. 565–572
17. "The Clock Ticks for 80,000 Americans," press release, National Kidney Foundation, May 2003.
18. "Facts-at-a-Glance," press release, National Kidney Foundation, April 2003.
19. "The Clock Ticks for 80,000 Americans," press release, National Kidney Foundation, May 2003.
20. Ian Williams, "China Sells Organs of Slain Convicts," *London Observer,* Dec. 10, 2000.
21. Francis Delmonico, M.D. et al., "Ethical Incentives—Not Payment—for Organ Donation," *New England Journal of Medicine,* vol. 346, no. 25, June 20, 2002, p. 2002

INDEX

Index

Index

Index